Thesis and Dissertation

Thesis and Dissertation

Sunil Chumber, Neerja Bhatla, Shyam S. Chauhan,
Ravinder Kumar Batra, Manoj Singh,
Parmod K. Bithal, Shashi Kant

PEEPEE

PUBLISHERS AND DISTRIBUTORS (P) LTD.

Thesis and Dissertation

Published by
Pawaninder P. Vij

Peepee Publishers and Distributors (P) Ltd.
Head Office: 160, Shakti Vihar, Pitam Pura
Delhi-110 034 (India)

Corporate Office: 7/31, Ansari Road, Daryaganj
Post Box-7243
New Delhi-110 002 (India)

Ph: 65195868, 23246245, 9811156083

e-mail: peepee160@yahoo.co.in

e-mail: peepee160@rediffmail.com

e-mail: peepee160@gmail.com

www.peepeepub.com

First Edition: **2007**

Reprint: **2009**

ISBN: 81-8445-029-X
978-81-8445-029-3

Printed at
Lordson, C-5/19, Rana Pratap Bagh, Delhi-110 007

Dedication

To Shishir and Kavita Vani, my parents, others that I have sacrificed for my own interests, my teachers and my colleagues, especially Peush, Anurag, Anita and Maneesh, past and present Residents of Surgery Unit I, especially Sanket, whose process of submitting the thesis protocol parallels the writing of this monograph, nurses and staff and patients, who cooperate with all of us in more ways than one, for the completion and success of many *theses* and *dissertations* and lastly animals (*I hope that it is correct to dedicate a monograph to animals*) that are studied and often sacrificed (*and remain unacknowledged*).

Sunil Chumber

To those who played a major role in shaping my thinking- my father, Joginder Nath Sikka, a great role model and visionary with a never-say-die attitude, who taught me the importance of discipline, integrity, clarity of thought and purpose. My father-in-law, Jagdish Chand Bhatla, a giant among men, who said to me when I was doing my thesis, "Do research that is new, path-breaking and meaningful". My mother, Mona Sikka, emphasised the need to play a meaningful role in society and encouraged me to achieve simply by believing in me. Mummy, Anil, Ameeta and Varun for their unstinted support. Akshay, Aditya and Rahul, whose outspoken comments keep me rooted in present-day reality. And, of course, generations of bright AIIMS students whose inquisitive, thought-provoking questions and discussions kept me on my toes. It's been a great journey.

Neerja Bhatla

I acknowledge the cooperation of my children-Vaibhav and Devashree and support of my wife Anista. I am also thankful to my M.Sc., M.D. and Ph.D students in helping me to learn enough so that I could contribute to this monograph.

Shyam S. Chauhan

I acknowledge and dedicate this work to my post-graduate students who have stimulated me to contribute towards the publication of this book.

Ravinder Kumar Batra

Teachers, students and family.

Manoj Singh, Parmod K.Bithal, Shashi Kant

Foreword

Research is a serious thing. It requires conceiving an idea or a hypothesis on a subject, followed by proper review of available knowledge in the literature in that area and its deficiency that needs further inquiry.

In higher medical education in the postgraduate level, undertaking a research project in the form of a *thesis or dissertation* is a mandatory exercise during the course of the Residency programme in most universities in India and abroad. In fulfilling this objective, a student has to acquire knowledge about methods of doing an inquiry in medical sciences. At times such an exercise in the form of a small epidemiological survey of a particular disease or problem in the society is given to a student even at the level of undergraduate courses during the summer among an attempt to create interest among MBBS students for doing research.

In this connection, a postgraduate student has to learn about research methodology and it being a difficult and new aspect to many students, requires guidance and supervision from the teacher. The guides/teachers have to provide such necessary inputs to the student through journal club discussion in the departmental teaching activities and also via Internet search, which has become a part of academic exercise for students as well as the teacher. Technology has today become an important tool of information dissemination in all branches of medical studies.

Any exercise in doing a research work and to produce quality research demands proper planning with sincerity and honesty and above all hard work with dedication and intelligent application of minds are needed during the course of work for producing a standard product. The guide or teacher supervising the work has to spend time in the laboratory or clinical situations with the student and the team of workers associated with the work, for achieving such a goal. *After all, research is a team work*! It requires suitable funding as well as ethical support from the institution/university, to meet the expenses of the project.

Everyday there is new information/knowledge emerging from various groups in the medical sciences, be it the basic aspect of medicine like genetics or molecular medicine and virology etc. or any clinical or epidemiological data. In India, there is ample opportunity for postgraduate students to do research in clinical medicine, as we have a large number of patients of different diseases or conditions. I believe that during a postgraduate course, the student can produce a great deal of research work under able guidance of the learned teachers. Research writing is also an art and any useful research work must be put into print media for diseemination of new knowledge and its clinical use in practice of medicine. Communication skills in writing is also important.

The book *Thesis and Dissertation* written by the authors will, I believe, go a long way in providing useful information and guidance to many students, while undertaking the work on a research project during his or her postgraduation courses. The authors have made sincere efforts to bring out various facets of doing research for a Resident doctor in this book and I hope, their efforts would benefit many.

Professor Ramesh C.Deka
Professor and Head of Otolaryngology and Dean
All India Institute of Medical Sciences, New Delhi

Contributors

Dr. Sunil Chumber
Additional Professor, Department of Surgical Disciplines, and Sub-Dean-Academics
All India Institute of Medical Sciences, New Delhi.

Dr. Neerja Bhatla,
Additional Professor, Department of Obstetrics and Gynecology, and former Sub-Dean-Academics
All India Institute of Medical Sciences, New Delhi.

Dr. Shyam S. Chauhan,
Professor, Department of Biochemistry
All India Institute of Medical Sciences, New Delhi.

Dr. Ravinder Kumar Batra,
Professor, Department of Anaesthesiology and Intensive Care
All India Institute of Medical Sciences, New Delhi.

Dr. Manoj Singh,
Professor, Department of Pathology
All India Institute of Medical Sciences, New Delhi.

Dr. Parmod K. Bithal,
Professor, Department of Neuroanaesthesiology
All India Institute of Medical Sciences, New Delhi.

Dr. Shashi Kant,
Professor, Centre for Community Medicine
All India Institute of Medical Sciences, New Delhi.

Preface

Submission of a *thesis* or *dissertation* is not only mandatory for completing a postgraduate course or acquiring a degree, but it is also a great opportunity to learn the basics of research methodology and publication–so vital in today's world. The components of a thesis involve writing a thesis protocol, a limited period of research and actual writing of thesis or dissertation, bringing it out in print form, submission to academic divisions of the institution and its evaluation by external examiners or its public defense as in the case of doctoral dissertations. A graduate who undertakes this difficult journey has few friends who will be able to help him; he may have research guides but he does not always have a sense of the direction that he must take. This short text is intended as a compass on this difficult journey.

From inception to completion, a Junior Resident has about 2 to 2½ years and a doctoral candidate has 3 to 5 years. This period has a way of flying by. This monograph can help to frame an academic calendar that will allow timely and smooth completion of your project.

We all hope that you will find these guidelines useful and wish you the best of luck for your successful writing of thesis and dissertation and your future academic life.

Authors

Message to Students

The journey of medical research is one marked by many obstacles and is often dreary and monotonous in which many a student is lost. Often the Guides are the only hope for such innocent travelers. For many years, the medical research was captive in the hands of major institutions. However, it is being increasingly recognized that this need not be so and medical research can often be conducted from not so well-recognized institutions or centers which are equipped with fewer facilities. In fact research for purposes of thesis and dissertations requires more of application of mind and less of tools and machinery.

Candidates in the process of preparing a thesis should be focused on their work and take their Guides into confidence at every step. The Guides too must devote adequate time to the candidate. Only a positive attitude will yield useful research worthy of publication and bring honors to candidate, Guides and institution.

I hope that this monograph will be the spark to ignite the minds of the students to conduct proper research and, even more importantly, to present it well.

Prof. Ravi Saksena,

Prof. and Head, Department of Anaesthesiology and Intensive Care Unit

All India Institute of Medical Sciences, New Delhi.

Research in the form of thesis and dissertation is an important component of post-graduate medical education in our country. For DNB programmes also, the candidates are required to submit thesis both for the Board as well as for the Superspecialities. In order to ensure thesis work of good quality, it is necessary that the candidates must have sound background of basic research concepts and also have skills in writing good thesis.

The present book is very comprehensive and would be valuable resource for the candidates while they are writing thesis protocol, planning collection of data and writing the final thesis. All the writers have vast experience and expertise in guiding post-graduate medical students and the way they have clarified the research related complex issues, is highly commendable.

The book will be a useful guide not only for the student but also for all consultants and medical personnel associated with post-graduate medical education and research.

Dr. A.K. Sood,
Executive Director,
National Board of Examinations,
New Delhi.

Research is undertaken when you conceive a novel idea about etiology, diagnosis or therapy and want to test its validity. In this endeavor you leave no stones unturned in unraveling the truth by conceiving a focused research question, conceptualizing the most appropriate research study design, with careful selection of patients, investigative tools and optional sample. Later, you sweat out in the conduct of research with collection of data without random errors and biases. The next step is painstaking statistical analysis of the data and preparation of the document.

Good thesis writing entails a comprehensive account of your project in a crisp and easily comprehensible language such that the reader is able to grasp the essence of the work without confusion.

It is the solemn duty of a good researcher to disseminate the knowledge obtained through his valid and reliable research. It is not enough to perform an extremely important research (usually with immense potential for human benefit) if the information is not published and spread among the potential users. Thesis should be regarded as the first formal and detailed publication of your research. This publication will also pave the way to expansion and exploration of your research hypothesis by further research by others. I wish you enjoy transcribing your research into your thesis.

Prof. Anurag Srivastava,
Department of Surgical Disciplines,
All India Institute of Medical Sciences, New Delhi.

Students are introduced to research work generally at the postgraduate level. During conduct of such research, students are expected to acquire essential skills of planning, executing (*psychomotor component*) and concluding the research work. There is always a knowledge (*cognitive*) component to execute psychomotor skills. Thus, the knowledge as to how to conduct research remains an important and major component of all such researches. All these factors determine how well you are going to conduct your research work.

The thesis is a window to all your efforts - which you have put in doing research and concluding it. My experience suggests that a large number of students do not put in their *will* and virtually consider their *thesis work* as *(un)necessary obligation*. However, there are several other factors, which make students think so—the medical fraternity needs to ponder over these factors.

The thesis is essentially considered as a student's product (some students feel so and boast of too), but in reality it is not so. The thesis is the product of joint effort of student and chief guide. Both the student and the chief guide are equally accountable for poor performance of *thesis work*. The chief guide should not forget that with his heavy work schedules and unavoidable commitments, the main research output of any institution lies on these young shoulders. The candidate requires guidance at the inception of protocol, conduct of the research, explanation of results and in a thorough check for midcourse corrections. Thus, the students can really do well if they devote their time after fully understanding the reasons of doing research.

I suggest that fresh students do require a beginner's course work before conducting thesis work. This may be done both at institutional level, departmental level and also at the level of research groups. The department may arrange interim thesis-presentation for the purpose of mid-course corrections. Frequent guide-student interaction is the most important factor in successful outcome of thesis research work. This book is going to be a boon for students and institution as well.

The book *Thesis and Dissertation* is written by the authors, who have all gone through all phases of postgraduate education. I consider the book as a guiding resource material to all budding researchers– a must have on this arduous research journey. I wish all candidates the best in thesis writing and in life.

Dr. KK Deepak
Prof. of Physiology and Sub-Dean (Examinations)
All India Institute of Medical Sciences, New Delhi.

Contents

Chapter 1

Introduction to Thesis and Dissertation

In most universities, research institutes and medical colleges, a thesis or dissertation is an integral part of all master's and doctoral degree programmes. In the case of M.D./M.S. and M.Sc., a dissertation is submitted in partial fulfillment of the requirements for the degree, but a Ph. D. is awarded solely on the basis of the thesis. In the monograph, dissertation and thesis have been used interchangeably and referred to as thesis. The thesis may take the form of a study, an experiment, a survey, or a project.

Purpose of the Thesis

The preparation of a thesis should develop in the candidate a broad understanding of current knowledge in the relevant field. This process should inculcate a scientific approach to research, i.e. identification of a research problem by a thorough survey of the literature, addressing the problem by performing relevant experiments, presenting the data in an understandable format, drawing meaningful conclusions from the results in the light of the existing knowledge and discussing these in the context of previously reported results in published literature.

General Nature of Thesis

The thesis serves to train students in the processes of scholarly inquiry and writing under the directions of members of the Faculty.

Generally, the candidate is assigned to a guide, who helps the candidate to select a topic for the thesis, includes members from related departments, and prepares the protocol. The protocol is approved by the Faculty of the Department and submitted to the Dean, who finally approves it for research. Once completed, the research work is summarized in the form of the thesis and submitted to the Dean, who then sends it to External Faculty for evaluation.

Candidates who have submitted a Thesis for their doctoral work have to defend the work at a *Public Defense* or *Oral Presentation*. The student, the chief guide, and the student's thesis committee are responsible for ensuring that the dissertation is presented in acceptable scholarly style and correct form.

The instructions in this guide intend to bring uniformity to *theses* and *dissertations* at the national level among Medical Colleges and at the National Board of Examinations, and generally apply to all disciplines. Although it is recognized that *theses* and *dissertations* from different departments or disciplines will exhibit some differences, certain requirements of format are common to all.

A variety of style manuals are available (see Bibliography and References) to assist students in writing a thesis. The guidelines in this manual include information on editorial style—the rules and guidelines necessary to ensure clear, consistent presentation of the printed work. Editorial style brings about uniformity in use of punctuations and abbreviations, construction of tables, selection of headings and citation of references, as well as many other elements that are part of every manuscript.

The minimum specifications described here must be met in order for a thesis to be accepted. The styles of earlier *theses* should ideally not be used as style and format models because they may not reflect current standards and requirements.

Chapter 2

Choosing a Topic and a Guide

Choosing a Topic/Subject for the Thesis

Generally, the topic or the subject for the thesis is allotted to the candidate by the Guide and/or Co-guides. This is often with the participation of other Faculty members from the same Unit, Department or allied Departments.

In Basic disciplines, it depends upon the focus of the laboratory because every area of research requires a particular set of instruments and laboratory facilities. Most often, an M.D., M.Sc. or Ph.D. student is given a part of an ongoing research project as a topic of his/her thesis. This arrangement not only ensures continuous support to the research student in terms of research facilities but may also provide financial assistance in the form of research fellowships, e.g., JRF, SRF, etc.

In clinical disciplines also, the topic may pertain to an area of the guide's interest. Rarely is a candidate asked to choose a topic for himself – in fact this may seem terrible to the candidate. If, however, there is some area that interests the candidate, he/she should not hesitate to say so. The subject of the thesis should be simple. It should be topical and preferably one of public health importance. It is easier and faster to do research on material easily available (e.g. inguinal hernia or chest infection) than on material that is uncommon or rare (e.g. endocrine pancreatic tumors or CML in children). A thesis on laparoscopic cholecystectomy can be finished in a year, whereas one on carcinoma of esophagus could take three to five years.

Hence, a candidate must choose a common topic/subject—material for which is easily available and one that can be finished in due time. Of course, a challenging topic when completed has its own rewards.

Allotment/Selection of a Guide

Generally, a candidate (i.e. you) is allotted to a Guide (it is not the other way round); only rarely will some departments ask you to choose your guide. This will invariably lead you to one of the *popular* guides. However, he may already have several candidates and, hence, no time for you!

Guides are allotted candidates by rotation. The same applies when there are several Units in a Department. Generally, a guide will be allotted a candidate, once in two years. Where there are more candidates, this allotment is more frequent. Senior Faculty members are allotted more candidates. At any given time, a Faculty member cannot be Chief guide of more than five Ph.D. students. Also, a Faculty member cannot be a Chief Guide if his/her retirement is due in less than three years.

Junior Faculty members, i.e. Lecturers and Assistant Professors, are more frequently co-guides on a thesis. Once they have experience of more than two or more years, they become eligible for allotment of thesis candidates independently. It is generally a good experience to be a candidate under such a young guide—(they may be willing to write your Protocol and do your thesis for you! However, this may not be such an advantage in the long run).

Whether by allotment or by selection, for the candidate, this marks the beginning of a new relationship(s)—nine out of ten will turn out to be very pleasant associations and will last a lifetime. For the one for whom the thesis has turned out to be an unpleasant affair, we have this to say to the candidate–you need to interact with your guide only for as long as the thesis is not written and submitted. Hence, complete your thesis fast and move on in life! Alas, instances of sexual harassment and suicides too have been known to be associated with thesis work! (Please do not hesitate to discuss these problems with the Head of your Department or the Academic/College Section, whose role is to protect your interests).

Lastly, it is not in the interest of a candidate to insist on doing a thesis with a particular guide only. The Department may not take to this kindly, especially if there is a policy of allotment of guides by rotation. It may also be embarrassing for the guide (how-so-ever flattering it may seem)!

Submission of Thesis Protocol

Thesis Protocol

The thesis protocol is an outline of the plan of study that details the research question, background and rationale for the study. It includes an introduction, a brief review of literature with references, the aims and objectives, materials and methods and the study proforma (see Fig. 3.1).

The candidate must select a topic and submit the thesis protocol within **three to four months** (or the specified time in your college/institution) from the date of joining the Master's programme. Ph.D. students, are given a period of **six months** after admission to submit their protocol. By this time, a candidate is expected to have performed preliminary experiments to ensure the feasibility of the study.

To plan a study, one must extensively survey the relevant literature and pinpoint the lacunae in the field. An appropriate study should then be planned to fill this gap. Since the normal duration of Ph.D. programme is up to five years, it involves more rigorous work as compared to M.D./M.S. and M.Sc. programmes.

The **last date** for submission of the Thesis Protocol for you is: ....
(enter the date in your own hand).

If submission of protocol is delayed beyond this date, your Residency programme will automatically be extended by 6 months and you will appear for your final Master's examination six months later. (If you are a female resident, who avails of maternity leave, then again the programme is extended by six months).

Title of Thesis

The title of the thesis should indicate the content as precisely and briefly as possible, e.g. *Effectiveness of Different Regimens in the Treatment of Lymphnode Tuberculosis: A Prospective, Randomized, Follow-up Study*. Do not use abstract terms in a title, or wordings that suggests a much broader scope than is actually covered, or gives an unclear or misleading impression.

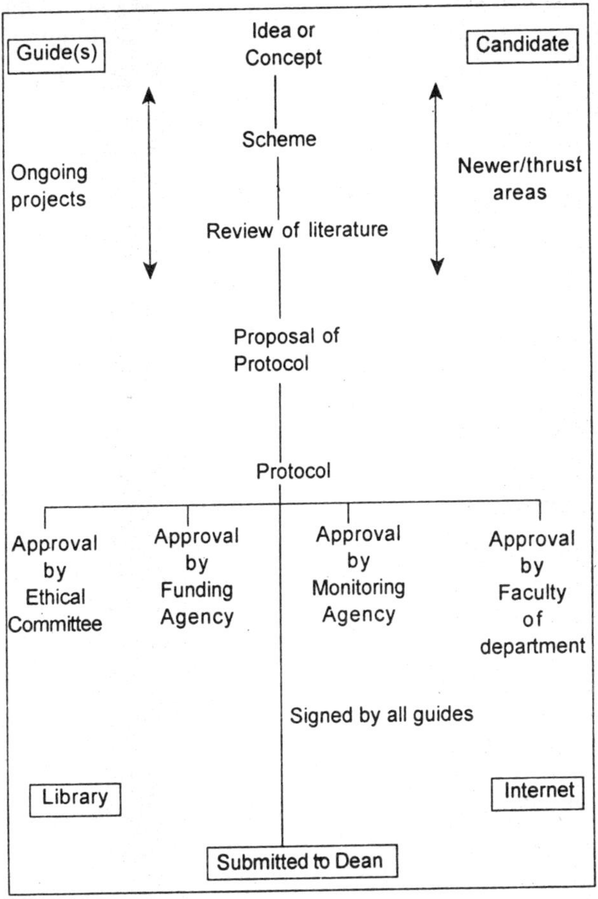

Fig. 3.1: Steps in development of thesis protocol

Some students find the title-subtitle form useful, e.g. *Primary Hyperparathyroidism: Neuro-psychiatric Manifestations Before and Following Surgery*. The title remains scholarly. It should **not** read like a sensational newspaper headline (e.g. *Sick in the mind? Get operated!*—This title and this form of title are not acceptable.)

The title of the thesis is either written in capital letters (uppercase) or first letter of every word except conjunctions are written in uppercase.

Scientific names of micro-organisms appearing in the title are either written in italics or underlined. In these, the first letter of the generic name (name of genus) is written in uppercase while the first letter of specific name (name of species) is written in lowercase, e.g., *Escherichia coli*. One should not use abbreviation(s) in the title.

Chief Guide—Co-guides

The Chief Guide generally decides who the other co-guides will be. The co-guides are usually from other departments who are required to assist in the research but, more importantly, to make facilities from their laboratories, etc. available for your research. Often, at least one of the Co-guides is included from the same department. This ensures continuity of your work in case your Guide is away on long leave, etc. It is always wise to include a co-guide with knowledge in Statistics if your Guide is not an expert in this area.

For Ph.D. degree at many centers, in addition to the Guide and Co-guides, a Doctoral Committee is constituted which monitors the progress of the work and suggests remedial measures if your research runs into rough weather. The doctoral committee is also empowered to recommend changes in the objectives of the thesis.

Planning a Research Project

We all want to write a thesis that produces valid results and is approved by our examiners (making us eligible for the specialty examinations for Master's). It must also be worthy of publication. To achieve these objectives we must begin with a well-designed study that will settle the *research question*. Sometimes all the criteria for designing a perfect study may not be met–but this does not necessarily mean that the work is without merit. Here, we will try to understand some basic aspects of research study design. The reader/researcher is referred to other texts for complete or advanced knowledge on research study design–for this is a subject in itself!

To design a good research project, the first ingredient is a proper work plan. It is necessary that one must be in frequent contact with the guides/supervisors and preferably a statistician or an epidemiologist. However, it is being made clear from the beginning that knowledge of statistics or even the most advanced computer program will not give results unless the study has been designed well right from the beginning. The principle of GIGO (Garbage In, Garbage Out) applies here as well. Let us try to understand a few things about our proposed research study/ project.

1. *The project must be feasible*!—This refers not only to resources (time and money), but also to whether there is agreement on the meaning of the research question and parameters that need to be measured.
2. *What is the problem*? *What do we wish to learn*? There must be a clear goal in mind. Framing a good research question is the first step towards good study design. A research topic should preferably *answer one question* at a time! There is no point in analyzing data from a study that

was not properly designed to answer the research question under investigation. For example *High incidence of Carcinoma Thyroid is seen in Persons of Northern States- A Pilot Study* is a poor research question. It could be improved as *Incidence of Carcinoma of Thyroid in Northern States—the Contribution of Iodine Deficiency*.

3. *The research project must be simple*: When undertaking a research project, one must preferably study two groups at once, if at all possible. When only two groups are being studied, the research question is sharply focused. When too many factors are studied simultaneously, it is often difficult to sort things out, especially when the factors are chosen haphazardly. A control group is important to improve validity of the study.
4. *Complete data entry and evaluation*: For the research project to yield a proper result, all relevant data must be collected. If a critical piece of data cannot be obtained or is missing, perhaps the study should not be undertaken. The purpose of the research too must be reflected on beforehand. Treatment protocols must be clearly identified. *Is there any point in studying the effects of nutritional supplementation in a population that is already healthy? Is it ethical to study an unhealthy population while denying them treatment?* Several of these queries must be reflected on before start of the research project.
5. *Research and responsibility*: Research is usually conducted with a view towards publication and dissemination. Hence, you must be aware of the possible consequences of your work as several public policies may be changed when particular results are reported in an improper manner or research may even come to a halt.

Methodology of Research

A few words on methodology of research may not be out of place at this point. Several issues are discussed in this section that pertain to designing of the research trial and subsequently to the writing the thesis itself. For detailed discussions, the readers are referred to other texts.

The purposes of writing this section on methodology of a research study are two folds:

1. To assist the examiner/reader to visualize the manner in which the research was conducted. If the reader can duplicate your work based on the methodology described by you, then this objective has been adequately achieved.
2. To assist the examiner/reader to evaluate the *Results and Conclusions* of the study on their own. The details provided in these sections should be of such nature and quantity that would allow the reader to form an opinion about the validity of your findings.

Word Count in Thesis

While writing for a journal that frequently has a cap on word count of the article, it may become difficult to achieve a balance between different sections of the write up. However, for purposes of writing a thesis, where we do not have constraint of space, it is better to err on the side of providing more information rather than less. Alas, this advice should not be misconstrued to provide detailed information on well-established procedures/ processes (as appendices/annexures) with the intention of making the thesis look bulky or scholarly!

The methodology section in the thesis should follow a logical sequence and be comprehensive in nature. The following points should be kept in mind regarding the planned research project while writing the Thesis Protocol/Thesis:

Study Area/Study Setting

A detailed description of prevailing conditions where the study was conducted helps the readers to understand the context in which to interpret the findings of the study. For example, if you were to conduct multi-drug resistant tuberculosis (MDR-TB) at a tertiary healthcare center such as at All India Institute of Medical Sciences or at a rural Primary Health Center, the results of the study are likely to be very different. The differences in the results are likely be due to the differences in patients' characteristics and the *referral bias* operating at the level of a tertiary care health centre.

This aspect of study design is especially important when the study is conducted at *field level*. It is not sufficient only to state that the study was carried out in a slum area or a resettlement colony. A paragraph on general socio-economic status of the population, literacy status and main occupation of the dwellers, the existing health facilities, and any other information that might have bearing on the study question should also be provided. For example, if a slum area has been adopted by a Non-Governmental Organization (NGO) or Governmental agency for literacy programme or income generation scheme, or any other such schemes that have a bearing on health status of the population, then a study conducted on malnutrition may be affected by these factors in a particular manner. Therefore, all such information should be provided in detail. If you have clearly characterized the setting of the study, the examiner/reader is in a better position to understand the results of the study in that context.

Study Period

The period of data collection should be clearly mentioned, as there may be a gap between the completion of study and its publication. Identification of the period in which the data collection has been carried out also helps the reader to pinpoint the time that the results of the study refer to.

Study Population

You should describe in detail the eligibility criteria for recruitment in the study. Explicit *inclusion* and *exclusion criteria* help to focus on the group to which the results of the study apply. You may also chose to exclude certain individuals based on age, sex, ethnicity, or any other personal or medical history. This exclusion simply means that the results of the study may not be applicable to the excluded group(s). Clear delineation of eligibility criteria also helps the examiner/reader to compare the results of your study with other studies that may or may not have the same restrictions for recruitment.

Sample Size

Usually a large number of eligible persons spread over a big geographical area are potentially available to be included in the study (*source population*). Obviously, it is neither possible nor desirable to include all of them in the study. Hence, we include only a small subset of all the available persons (*study population*). Intuitively, we all know that if we were to take only a small number of subjects (study population) from all available eligible study subjects (source population), then we may not be able to generalize the results to the source population. Alternatively, we could include everyone in the source population and thus eliminate the need of generalization altogether. However, this approach would be most *cost-inefficient* way of performing research. Hence, a balance has to be arrived at wherein the number of subjects included are sufficient enough to provide the answers that we are looking for and yet are no more than what is absolutely necessary. Thus, the concerns of *cost-efficiency* as well as *validity* of the study findings are addressed simultaneously.

The sample size can be calculated using standard formulae before undertaking the study. Depending upon the study design and the research question, the required size of sample may differ. The information required to calculate the sample size is:

a. Expected prevalence of the disease condition in the population
b. The Confidence level desired by the researcher (e.g. C.I. of 95%)
c. The relative (or absolute) precision of the estimate required by the researcher and
d. Magnitude of the effect considered as clinically relevant.

It is wise to take help of a Statistician/Epidemiologist while preparing the Thesis Protocol. The details of sample size calculation too should be incorporated in the Thesis Protocol. At the very least, mention should be made about the *research assumptions* and the *formulae* employed for calculation of sample size. Many a times the required sample size is so large that it is not practically feasible to study it in the time frame available to the Resident for a thesis. In such a situation, the sample size for purposes of the thesis should be explicitly mentioned. The sample size to be studied would also depend upon the *logistics* and *availability of study subjects* and other *time constraints*.

Sampling Procedure

Once it has been decided that some rather than all of the source population will be recruited for the research project, then the next issue is how to select the sample?

The method by which the subset is selected from a larger pool is called sampling procedure. There are several ways of performing the sampling. The adequacy and appropriateness of sampling has the greatest impact on the validity of results of the study. If the samples are chosen inappropriately, they might provide result that are *internally valid* but cannot be generalized to any other population, i.e. are not *externally valid.* In this section of your thesis, you must also try to convince your examiner/reader that the selection process was not influenced by the personal preferences (*selection bias*) of the researcher(s). You must also document that adequate measures were adopted to eliminate selection bias.

The calculation of sample size also takes into account the sampling procedure. This calculation is based on the assumption that sampling is on random basis. Hence, documenting the sampling procedure too would assure your examiner/reader that the sample size is adequate.

Tools

The tools or instruments used for measurement or data collection should be described in detail e.g. if Salter's scale was used for weighing, then one should describe the maximum weight that can be measured by it as well as the least count. The same information should also be provided if bathroom scale was used instead for purposes of weighing.

The questionnaire and interview schedule are also study instruments. If a standard and published tool was used then it should be mentioned and reference provided. In case *adaptation* was made to suit the local conditions, then the same should be described. It is a good idea to provide the *sensitivity* and *specificity* of the instrument being used. In case you are translating a standard tool into local language for the purpose of the study, clearly state the process adopted by you to ensure that the translation is valid. If the details of the tools are too long, it can be added as appendices/ annexure.

Variables

Explicit mention should be made of variables under study to help the examiner/reader to understand the key components of the study. Some researchers also prefer to state the projected *primary* and *secondary outcome measures*. The sample size is often calculated keeping in mind the primary outcome measures. A clear definition of signs, symptoms, and disease under consideration should be made to avoid any later misunderstandings.

Operational Definition

For purposes of a research study, it is best to employ definitions that are used widely and have international acceptance. This allows you to make comparisons with the work carried out by other researchers. If a standard or widely accepted definition does not exist, then you may think of using an *operational* definition. This definition should be based on prevailing circumstances that are specific to your research study. Operational definitions should only be a measure adopted as a last resort.

Study Design

You may choose to observe and document an event and let nature take its own course. Such a study would be an *observational study*. However, if you were to intervene in any manner in the ongoing processes and then record and report your findings, it would be called *experimental study*. The observational studies are of two types - one can have *descriptive study* and *analytical study*. In descriptive study, the condition, disease or heath status of interest is described without any attempt to find associations or a putative cause. A *case study* and *case series* are examples of descriptive studies. However, when attempt is made to find an association between the disease status and exposure to a particular stimulus, then such design is called analytical study. An analytical study could be *ecological study*, *cross-sectional study*, *case-control study* or *cohort study*.

The unit of study in ecological study is the entire population or a large sub-group of the population. Correlation is made between a disease status and another factor that is considered as the cause e.g. trends in tobacco production and lung cancer mortality. In an ecological study, the data is usually generated for some other purposes; whereas the generation of data is often easy, but the interpretation of the result should be performed most cautiously.

A *cross-sectional study* is also known as a *prevalence study* because it measures the prevalence of a disease or health event in the population. This may be *point prevalence* or *period prevalence study*. Point prevalence has often been likened to a snapshot wherein the situation as it existed at a given point of time is captured. The time frame is kept to a minimum in point prevalence. If the time period is extended the design is then called period prevalence study. The exposure and the outcome are measured at the same time. Hence, it may become difficult to ascertain the temporality of the event. The causal inference in this study design is usually weak, but due to ease of carrying out and being relatively economical, cross-sectional studies are quite common.

Case-control study: This study design is most suited for uncommon or rare diseases. In this a group of patients with the disease called *cases* are identified and studied. A comparable group without the disease status is called *controls*. The rate of occurrence of the putative cause in both the group is compared to ascertain its *role as a causative agent*.

Theoretically, the study design is simple. However, in practice, several difficulties arise during the conduct of the study. The cases included should represent *all* cases that occur in the population. If you are conducting research at a tertiary care centre, then it is probable that only cases with *certain* characteristics may be recruited. This is due to referral bias. If only prevalent cases were included, then those that die in the *initial rapid death phase* of the disease would be missed out from the study. Similarly, the controls or control cases should represent the exposure level prevalent in the community from where these cases come from. Most often controls are recruited from the hospital setting. This may be advantageous for the Candidate but there are several disadvantages of this form of recruitment as well.

Cohort study design: In a cohort study design we start with healthy people and follow them up for certain period of time to assess the occurrence of disease or health-event of interest. The exposure status of this population is known as opposed to case-control study design where the disease or outcome of interest has already taken place and we subsequently measure the exposure status. If the time lag between exposure to the stimulus and occurrence of disease is long then one can derive information from *historical cohort* e.g. as the exposure of patients to asbestos and development of lung cancer is long, one can revert to available records and assemble a group of persons who were working in coal-mines, about twenty years back, and treat them as a cohort. This is also referred to as *retrospective cohort study design*. If the cohort is constructed afresh and followed up in future, it is described as *prospective cohort study design*. The cost of conducting this type of study is a major constraint in research.

The experimental studies consist of randomized controlled trials, field trials, and community trials. *Randomized controlled trials* are used to compare new preventive or therapeutic regimens. In this, the basic design is to enroll eligible participants and randomly allocate them to either control group or treatment group. In fact there could be more than one treatment group and simultaneous comparison with control group can be performed. To make the study groups similar, a *placebo* is sometimes used in control arm of the study design.

Blinding is carried out in the allocation groups to minimize the *bias*. When only the participant is blinded it is *single-blind*, when the researcher too is also blinded, it is called *double-blind*, and when, in addition, the data analyst is also blinded it is called as *triple-blind* study design.

Field trials are conducted among apparently healthy individuals residing in the community. The data is thus collected in the field. The purpose of a field trial is to test if a given medical intervention among healthy yet *at risk* population is able to reduce the risk of disease. For example children in community may be healthy but at risk for developing diseases. Hence, a new vaccine, when introduced is first field-tested to see if it able to reduce the risk of disease among children. Again, cost is a major concern in the design of a field trial.

Community trial is a study design where the whole community is treated as a single group. Since, many diseases have their origin in social conditions, intervention at community level is required to overcome these diseases. In such situations, community trials may be undertaken. Research studies on cardiovascular diseases that are multifactorial in origin and having a strong social component could be one example for community trials. The problem with this study design is that random allocation to different groups cannot be performed. It is also difficult to get a comparison with another community where no intervention has been carried out and which can serve as a control group. Changes that may occur over period of time, that are independent of intervention, are often difficult to assess and to account for.

Data Collection, Storage, and Management

It is necessary to mention the software that was employed for data entry. Sometimes double data entry is resorted to when fidelity of data is of utmost importance. Since privacy of data is implicit and often explicit, one must also state the procedures adopted for securing the data and maintaining the confidentiality of the information. The statistical tests employed in compiling the *Results and Analyses* should be detailed and if statistical software was used then a complete reference of the same should be provided.

Ethical Consideration

Issues related to ethical practices in research are discussed in a separate section. The Final Thesis should mention that the Institutional Review Board has cleared the undertaken study.

Consent of the Participants

When recruiting patients for a research study, it is essential to have informed written consent from the study participants or subjects. The consent form should be in a language that is understandable to the study participants. The consent form should be read out for those participants who are illiterate and this should be attested by another person who acts as a witness. Consent for inclusion of children or mentally challenged persons should be obtained from parent(s) or legal guardian. A copy of the information that was provided or read to the participants as well as a copy of the consent form should be attached to the thesis as an appendix/annexure. If any compensation was offered to the participants it should also be declared.

Discussion

When completing the *Discussion* section, the results of your study should be compared and contrasted with other similar studies. If the findings are similar then one could comment that your findings are in agreement with those of other authors. However, do *not* panic if your findings are in disagreement with the studies of other researchers. You may have stumbled upon something that is truly important! In this section you must try to provide possible reasons for the observed differences.

Limitations

The findings of the study should be evaluated for alternative explanations before concluding that the disease condition observed is the result of exposure to a particular agent. Alternative explanations to the available results may lie in *chance*, *bias*, and *confounding*.

Chance: Since we carry out research on a sample rather than the entire source population, the obtained result could be purely due to *luck of the draw*. The adequacy of sample size will determine the extent of role of chance. In addition, we should use statistical methods to calculate the Confidence Interval (CI).

Confidence interval is a range of estimate within which the true value of the finding would lie with a given certainty. This certainty is usually taken to be 95%. It means that even then, in one in twenty times the true value(s) would lie outside the calculated range.

Bias: Errors can vitiate any research study. If errors occur in random manner, then in the long run, they tend to *cancel-out* each other and the findings of the study is not skewed in any particular direction. Random errors tend to obliterate or diminish true association, if one exists. However, *bias* is a systematic error.

Bias leads to an incorrect estimate of association between exposure to a stimulus and disease. The types of bias can be classified into two groups i.e. selection bias, and measurement bias. *Selection bias* refers to systematic error in the way study participants were recruited whereas *measurement bias* refers to error in ascertaining the information from those recruited.

Unlike chance, bias cannot be quantified by statistical methods. The best way to deal with bias is to anticipate it and remove it during the design stage of the study. This requires good familiarity with the subject of the proposed study. Hence, it is important that a good review of literature is carried out during writing of the Thesis Protocol itself. While providing alternative explanations to your results, you should document the likelihood of bias in your study and the manner/direction in which your results would be affected if this bias had taken place.

Confounder: While one is trying to measure the association between exposure and the disease, it is possible that there exists another variable that has neither been controlled nor measured but which has a role to play in the observed association. Such a variable is called a confounder. It might fully or partially account for the observed association. The hallmark of a confounder is that it is associated with the exposure but independent of the exposure it is risk factor for the disease. Age and sex are the commonest confounders. The three ways to deal with confounders in a research study are randomization, restriction, and matching.

Randomization: This allocates known as well as unknown confounders into different groups purely on chance basis. Hence, the confounders are distributed in equal amounts to different study sub-groups and, hence, cancel-out each other. For this process to succeeded, the numbers should be sufficient to avoid chance imbalance between groups. Randomization can be as simple as assigning treatment by flipping a coin (not recommended!), assigning by odd and even numbers (also not recommended) or by consulting a randomization table or generating one at an internet site called www. randomization.com (preferred scientific methods). In general, randomization should be performed by someone not directly concerned with the study.

It should be ensured that randomization is not unethical. Subjects in the study cannot be randomized to a group that would undergo a harmful treatment or be knowingly given harmful or even *less than* optimum treatment.

Restriction: Another method to deal with confounder is to have a strict criterion of eligibility. For example, if race and sex are the potential confounders, then one could restrict the study to white males. Obviously, it would impinge upon the generalizability since the results could not be extrapolated to non-white or females.

Matching: This is yet another strategy to deal with confounding. In this strategy, the potential confounder is purposely distributed equally among the different sub-groups. Again the role of the confounder is nullified due to equal distribution among groups. One must however be careful in using appropriate statistical tools for analysis of matched study design data.

Writing the Protocol

Once the subject/topic and guides have been decided, it is time to write down the protocol. It is written in the following manner:

	No. of Pages
Title of Thesis Protocol	1
Name of Candidate, Guide and Co-guides	1
Introduction	1-2
Review of Literature	1-5
Aims and Objectives	1
Materials and Methods	1-3
References	1
Appendix- Proforma for the study	1-5
Total number of pages	8-15

Review of Protocol by Departmental Faculty

Once the Protocol is prepared, it is circulated to members of the Departmental Faculty for review and opinion. This is carried out by the Guide. The Faculty, after reviewing the Protocol, will write their comments. In some departments, a formal presentation may be made by the candidate or the guide to the entire Faculty or Department. This system of peer review and validation encourages healthy debate and improves the quality of the protocol by plugging any loopholes (of course, this also carries the danger of bringing out into the open, the differences between the Faculty).

Once accepted, i.e. after the suggestions made by the Faculty have been incorporated, the Final Protocol (2 or more duly signed copies) is sent to the Dean.

Chapter **4**

Carrying Out Research

After registration, a Ph.D. student gets a maximum duration of 5 years for submitting the thesis. The first six months out of this period are spent in choosing a laboratory and submission of a protocol after performing preliminary experiments and the last six months are available for writing the thesis. The remaining four years in between should be dedicated for the actual research work, communicating results and presenting your work in conferences.

For MD/MS students, this portion of the thesis work is carried out during nearly 2 years available to you from the time of submission of the thesis protocol till the last date for submission of thesis.

The Residents and researchers are advised in their own interest that they make a work plan in a manner that the bulk of the work, including the writing, is completed within the allotted time. The first two sections of the thesis, i.e. Introduction and Review of Literature can be drafted even before the work is completed.

The candidate is expected to read extensively on the topic of his research and look up at least the essential literature before he starts work on the project and interpreting the results. Subsequently, literature reviews should be carried out periodically so that one is abreast of all new information pertaining to the task at hand.

Estimate of the Total Amount of Work

It is a good idea to get a proper estimate of the work. If you are dealing with patients, then you can follow the method given on next page.

Number of patients included in your protocol: 50
Number of patients reported in one year: 35

This effectively means that if you are alert, you can finish the *work* of the thesis in less than two years time. However, if the number of patients attending the hospital is 25 per year, then you cannot afford to miss even one patient. If the number of patients attending the hospital is still lower, you will need to visit other hospitals to get additional patients to complete the thesis. These rough estimates are to ensure that all is going well and on schedule. What happens if you or your Guide falls ill or he/she goes abroad for two years? The candidate should be able to continue the work even in these circumstances. A second Co-guide from the department is invaluable in such a situation!

If you are working in the laboratory, then you must divide your work in such a manner that you have 20-30 % time available to take care of any delays or untoward incidents. If you are working on animals, then plan your work in consultation with your guides. This will require special clearances from specific committees. This is discussed in a later chapter.

Work done per month = n/20 (n = no. of cases)
Time to write the thesis = 4 to 6 months

Completing your Thesis Cases

Discipline is the essence of success! Be regular in doing your thesis. All your work on the cases should finish in 18 to 20 months time. This will give you about 4 to 6 months to write your thesis and submit on time.

It is a good idea to take help from your colleagues in doing your work. If you are out of town, ask them to work-up your cases and to keep records. It is also appropriate that you inform your guides that you are absent for this period and are returning at this particular time. Then, they are responsible for keeping track of your work.

If in a particular period, you are not able to do your cases, then you must contact your guides to discuss the reasons for this. If there are genuine reasons, then your guides could reduce the number of cases required. (However, this will require the Dean's consent).

Rotation Postings

During your Residency, you will be regularly rotated through other Departments as part of your Specialist's training. This cannot and should not be avoided nor should the postings be altered for your thesis work. In any case, your Department will not permit this.

This is again the time to contact your friends and ask them for help. They will help to keep track of your cases, work up your patients, help in their sampling and operations and help in maintaining their records. Of course, it also means that you will do the same for them!

Sometimes, your senior friends will ask you to dig out some references for them from the depths of the library. Please do not refuse to help them. This is a part of the same *give and take* – and this is how several candidates can do their thesis even when on Rotation Postings. You must also keep your guides informed about your postings.

There is no rotation for Ph.D., M.Sc. and M.D. students in disciplines of basic research.

Tabulating Data

It is a good idea to work-up your cases and enter them on a master chart on the same day itself. This ensures that you have a clear estimate of how your work is progressing and how much more needs to be done. This also ensures that you can analyze your data speedily. Some candidates will enter the data on a computer programme. However, *one hard copy must be retained* in case of data corruption or data loss.

Meeting your Guides

One must be regular in meeting the guides to apprise them of the work done, results obtained as well as difficulties encountered. These meetings should be held at least once a month. You must also apprise your guides regularly of the cases that you have performed. Only then can they help you to solve any problems that may arise. Mark these appointments on your schedules and make sure that they are marked on your Guides' schedules too!

Sometimes, you have nothing new to report-then also you are advised to meet your Guides – you may pick up a few tips that may prove useful in later life.

Also, you must regularly review literature and recent publications on the Internet to keep abreast of recent developments in literature.

Holding Doctoral Committee (DC) meetings at regular intervals also helps Ph.D. students in smooth running of their project.

Presenting in Conferences

Even while your research is being completed, you should present it in conferences. By presenting your work in conferences, you may not only get the opinion of other scientists working in this field but also get an opportunity to discuss about your problems. Thus, in a conference, you often find the solution to some of your wexing problems. In a conference, you may also find valuable material to complete some aspects of your work e.g. special reagents.

Publication of your Work

It is also strongly suggested that you communicate your results to a scientific journal as and when you have enough data for publication. *This is your bounden duty!*

Chapter 5

Thesis Writing

By this time you have already completed almost two years of your Residency or about 4 years if you are a Ph. D. candidate and are ready to write your thesis. If you have completed longer than this, then you are already late in reading this section. However, still carry on.

First of all, write down the last date for submission of the thesis below.

Today's date:...
Last date for submission of thesis:.....................................
Number of days left till deadline for submission of thesis:...days.

This gives you a rough estimate of the time left with you in an *academic do-or-die* situation. The writing of the thesis should be started immediately and completed and submitted at the earliest. Only these can be your immediate goals.

Do remember that the thesis is one of the essential criteria to fulfill so that you are eligible to appear for the Final Master's Examination.

No Thesis = No Examination

If you are a doctoral candidate, you get nothing if you do not complete your thesis.

Hence, buck up and start with the writing of the thesis at once (see Figures 5.1 and 5.2).

Collecting the Data

Writing of the thesis is started by locating the Thesis Protocol, collecting all the data and putting all the papers into a single file. This will be the eye-opening moment for you. You will suddenly

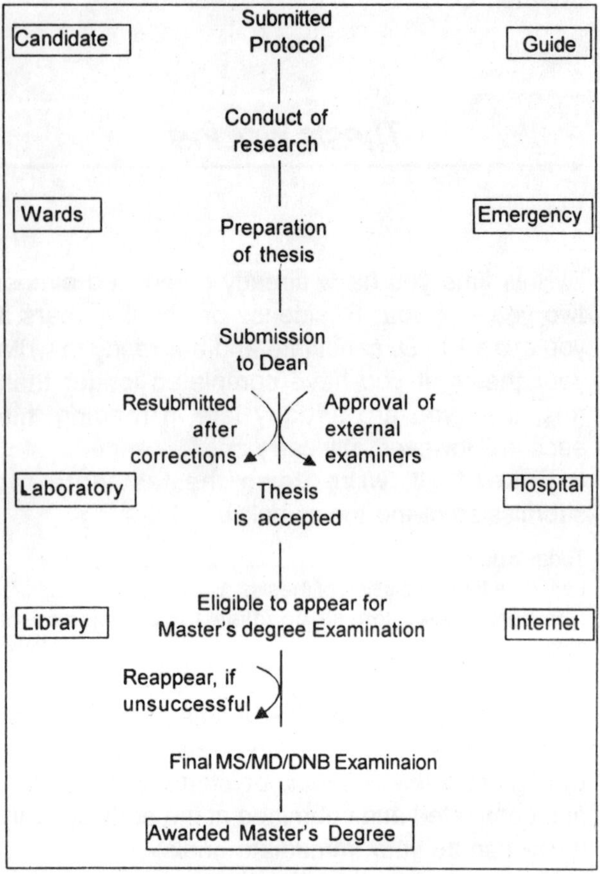

Fig. 5.1: Steps in preparation and submission of dissertation and outcome

realize exactly how much work still needs to be done and how little time you have to accomplish the same. This is a good time to refresh the Thesis Protocol, visit your Guides, go through the data and...

Locate the Library!

Hopefully this would have been done long, long ago. But perhaps some of you have been too busy with your duties, studies and research and have restricted your reading to the Internet. So now is the time to visit the local Library (As the song goes, it's now or never...). You will be spending the next

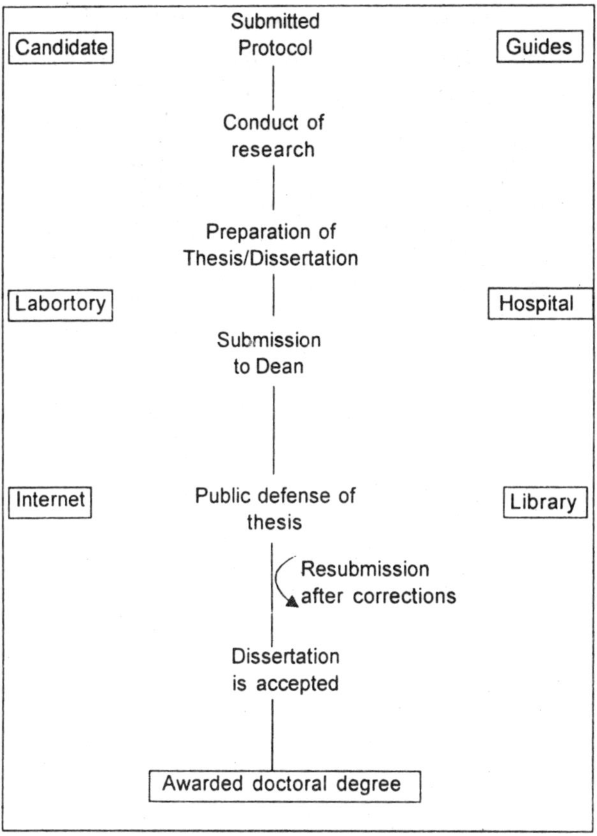

Fig. 5.2: Steps in preparation and submission of doctoral thesis and outcome

several weeks in this Library and soon it will seem like a second home to you.

At All India Institute of Medical Sciences, New Delhi, the B.B. Dixit Library is prominently located and is open 24 hours a day. Other candidates will locate the libraries in their respective colleges or cities and start allotting adequate time for reading the relevant literature. The National Medical Library is located in New Delhi on the Ring Road and is accessible to all for looking up recent references. Many of you will need to visit this library at some time in relation to your thesis and research since it contains several books and journals not available at the best college libraries. Try not to come during the season of thesis writing (but at this point you don't have any choice) and be very clear about what you want from this library. Make a list before you enter the library. If you are coming from out of town for finding references, please give adequate time for this process—it cannot be finished in one day.

The B.B.Dixit Library is an excellent library but not accessible to all. So it is a good time to look up your old friends at All India Institute of Medical Sciences. Another library that is of use, especially to students in basic research, is the Central Science Library in Delhi University at Maurice Nagar, Delhi.

Computer Facility

The Computer Facility services when available are useful for searching the Internet for references and email facility. Again, you must make a list of what you want before you start surfing e.g. keywords, authors, review articles, etc. Other students may have to resort to searching in Internet Cafes near their colleges—these are equally viable and cost-effective options.

Getting your own Computer/Internet

It is a good idea to get your own computer, Internet connection and printer while you are in the process of writing your thesis. Even the laptop range of computers has become cheap in India—hence a Resident can afford one now. You can also consider pooling your resources with other Residents who are finishing their theses at the same time!

Collecting Articles/References

It is expected that a Research Scholar will keep reading and collecting relevant literature during the entire course of study. For this purpose, it is preferable to devote a certain number of hours to the thesis every week. It is up to you to assess how much this period will be. Generally, two to three hours per week (outside your duties) will be enough for this work. During this period, you must visit the library and read up new journals. Make a photocopy of the required articles. Check on old journals for relevant articles. Keep all the relevant literature in a single file marked "Review of Literature". All these articles will be useful at the time of writing the thesis. Mark these visits to the library on your schedules now itself!

Progression of Work

It is important to keep track of the progress of your work. A method to monitor the rate of progression of your work is shown below:

Month 1	=	n/20 of work
Month 2	=	n/20 +n/20= 2n/20
Mon..		
Month 20	=	20n/20 = this means that all the required number of cases have been recruited.
Month 21	=	completion of Introduction and Materials and Methods.
Month 22	=	completion of Review of Literature, compilation of Results and Analysis.
Month 23	=	completion of Discussion, inclusion of all corrections made by Guides, preparation of tables, illustrations and photographs.
Month 24	=	completion of Thesis, signing of Final Thesis by Guides, submission of Thesis.

Where some candidates are concerned, the work of the last five months is unfortunately condensed into one month. This becomes extremely painful for the Guides–candidates are always chasing them at odd hours, painting them in a bad light and making them sacrifice their own work, families, vacations and other students!

The Guide can find little time for review of the work and cannot devote adequate time to help in the corrections. Sometimes, the guide has to attend to two or even three candidates in the same schedule (*and same deadlines*). All of this can be avoided if the candidate can stick to the above schedule. If you want to bring out a good thesis– give your Guide more time than you will give the printer or the binder!

Advice for the candidates:

1. Do not bring thesis at the last moment!
2. Give adequate time to guides for checking the thesis!
3. Get the progress of your research reviewed on regular basis.
4. Start writing *Review of Literature* during progress of research.
5. Do not *cut and paste* from original articles, internet sites and textbooks!

Chapter 6

Format of Thesis

Presently, there is no officially prescribed format for the thesis among various colleges in the country. However, the most commonly used format is discussed below and this is acceptable as a uniform standard for all theses in India. Several other formats are available and followed in other countries—for these, the student may check on the Internet or other books.

One of the aims of this manual is to bring about uniformity in thesis formats/manuscripts submitted by students from various disciplines. Theses written in past years are available in the B.B.Dikshit Library at All India Institute of Medical Sciences, or in the libraries of other Medical Colleges but, as discussed earlier, these should not be used as the reference standard as they often do not follow a clear style.

Paper and Printing

The paper used for the thesis must be *pure* white and of very good quality. The same brand and weight of paper must be used throughout the thesis. The commonly used paper for printing the thesis is A-4 sized photocopier paper. The dimensions of this paper are 8¼ x 11½ inches. The original manuscript must be typed or printed on *one side of the paper only.* Students may print ONE final copy directly from the inkjet or laser printer and make photocopies (also of very good quality). The print or type must have a consistent sharpness, clarity, and darkness throughout the text.

Fonts

Students should decide on a font style in the early stages of thesis preparation itself. This will help to avoid later changes in text alignment. All headings should have the same font style, all subheadings will have the same font style and the main text will have a third font style. The same font is to be used throughout the thesis, whether in preliminary pages, text, tables and figure captions, reference/bibliography pages, appendices, or page numbers.

The font size may either be 12 or 14, depending on the font chosen. The size should be large enough to make it easy for the reader (especially keeping in mind that examiners are usually presbyopic!). There can be no changes in the font (typeface) anywhere in the text.

Some commonly used fonts appropriate for your thesis are illustrated (see Table 6.1)., Verdana, Helvetica and Arial are the *sans serif* type of fonts.

Table 6.1: Commonly employed type fonts in the thesis

a. Times New Roman—A quick brown fox jumped over the lazy dog.
b. Courier—A quick brown fox jumped over the lazy dog.
c. Arial—A quick brown fox jumped over the lazy dog.
d. Helvetica—A quick brown fox jumped over the lazy dog.
e. New Century Schoolbook—A quick brown fox jumped over the lazy dog.
f. Bookman—A quick brown fox jumped over the lazy dog.
g. Palatino—A quick brown fox jumped over the lazy dog.
h. Geneva—A quick brown fox jumped over the lazy dog.
i. Verdana—A quick brown fox jumped over the lazy dog.

Formating

The format of the pages of the text should contribute to the continuity for the reader. Partially filled pages of text are not acceptable, except at the end of a chapter, or where there is insufficient room to place four or five lines of text either before or after a table.

The text is printed so that each page is filled from the top margin to the bottom. However, the bottom margin should be adjusted to avoid *widows* and *orphans*. A *widow* is a single initial line of a new paragraph at the bottom of the page, and an *orphan* is a single terminal line of a paragraph at the top of a page. In other words, a single line of a paragraph is not acceptable at either the top or bottom of a page.

Throughout the thesis, leave TWO spaces after punctuation at the end of a sentence. Do not hyphenate words at the end of a line except in the case of a compound word.

Any additions to the text of *foreign alphabets*, *scientific formulae*, or other *signs* that are not available on the keyboard or *Symbols* section in Microsoft Word (this must be rare indeed!), must be made with a fine-pointed art pen in permanent black ink. These are available in Microsoft Word in 'insert' 'symbols'.

Margins

Standard page size for a thesis is 8¼ × 11½ inches (A4 size paper). The following are the margins for the page. The left margin is wider to facilitate binding:

Left margin (binding edge)	1½ inches
Right margin	1 inch
Top margin (first line of text)	1 inch
Bottom margin	1¼ inches

The top margin is measured from the top edge of the page to the top of the first line. The bottom margin is measured from the bottom of the last line of type to the bottom edge of the paper. Margin requirements must be followed for photographs, figures, graphs, and appendices. ONLY page numbers should appear in the bottom margin. *Lastly, do justify lines.*

Spacing

Text: Only **double-spacing** is to be used throughout the manuscript.

Reference material: Single-spacing is to be used when writing the legends to figures and in the references. The reference material is single-spaced within each reference and double-spaced between references. The first line of each reference is flush with the left margin. Single spacing is also used in the following situations:

- When lines of chapter titles or subheadings are more than half a line in length, they may be divided, preferably using an inverted pyramid format, and single-spaced.
- Two-line headings and figure captions may also be single-spaced.

If there are two tables or figures on the same page, separate them by a triple-space. (A triple-space means 3 single-spaced blank lines or 2 double spaces).

Table numbers should be either chapter-based, i.e. Table 1.1, Table 2.3, Table 2.4, etc or should be in continuation throughout the thesis, e.g. Table 1, Table 2, Table 3, etc.

Corrections

Corrections that have been made by the guides or by you on the preliminary drafts must always be incorporated on the computer itself. If you are doing the work on a typewriter (very unlikely now!) then these corrections must be made in the original and must be done with attention to neatness. All text on the computer must be spell-checked before the printing. It is unpardonable to have white correction fluid on the final thesis or finished corrected copies. **No corrections with pencil or pen are permitted on the Final Thesis.** Hence, careful proofreading must follow any changes. Most colleges and their Academic

Sections would not accept these - even if you have managed to get them past the blind guides.

Page Numbering (Pagination)

Each page in a thesis must be assigned a number. Numbering is done in the following manner:

Preliminary Pages: The pages in the preliminary material must be numbered consecutively with lower case Roman numerals (e.g., ii, iii, iv, etc.). *Page numbers are placed in the lower margin, 1 inch from the bottom edge of the paper.*

Preliminary pages such as Abstract, Acknowledgments, Dedication, Abbreviations, Table of Contents, List of Tables, and List of Figures are numbered with the lower case Roman numerals in consecutive order.

a. **Title Page:** Only the **title page** does not bear any number even though it is considered as page i.
b. **Thesis Certificate:** The thesis certificate page is ii and is so numbered.
c. **Abstract Page:** An abstract of the entire work should be summed up in 300 words and placed here. The abstract page is page iii.

Text pages: All text pages must be numbered in the bottom margin 1 inch from the bottom edge of the paper using Arabic numbers. The Arabic numbers begin with the first page of Introduction (or Chapter I) and continue throughout the study, references, and appendices.

On pages printed in *landscape*, the page number should be placed in the same position as on the other pages.

All page numbers must be of the same typeface and type size as the text of the paper.

All page numbers stand-alone! No brackets! No punctuations!

Layout of the Thesis

The Thesis is set in the following order:

1. Title page
2. Certificate page (also a Signature page)
3. Abstract page
4. Dedication (optional)
5. Acknowledgments
6. Abbreviations page (optional)
7. Table of Contents
8. List of Tables
9. List of Figures
10. Introduction
11. Aims and Objectives
12. Review of Literature
13. Materials and Methods
14. Results and Observations (Analysis)
15. Discussion
16. Summary
17. Conclusions
18. List of References/Bibliography
19. Appendix
20. Copyright page (optional)
21. Master chart

Preliminary Pages

Abstract Page

Every thesis should contain an abstract. For some unknown reason, this practice is not uniformly followed—some departments insist on it but others not requiring this at all. The abstract should present an account of the thesis that will enable a reader to determine the necessity (or desirability) of reading the entire work. It should be well organized and brief but complete. The maximum length of the abstract is 300 words and it should be contained on a single page only (this is preferable). The count is taken word for word (the easy method, of course, is to let the computer do the word count). Style standards for the thesis also apply to the abstract.

The page of the abstract should be headed by the word "ABSTRACT" typed in all capitals, centered between margins. The text begins a double space below, is single-spaced, and is typed in normal paragraph form. The first word of each paragraph should be indented consistent with the rest of the paper. Although the abstract may have several paragraphs, it should contain no subtitles, paragraph headings, or citations. *The abstract precedes the thesis.* It is not included in the Table of Contents.

Dedication (Optional)

The dedication is brief. It appears immediately after the Abstract page and is numbered using lower case Roman numerals. A heading on this page is optional. When used, it is centered in all capitals. The text begins a double space below the heading.

Acknowledgements (Optional)

It is customary (although not obligatory) to acknowledge with gratitude individuals and organizations that have helped in the production of the thesis. It is correct to acknowledge the guides, colleagues and other persons who have helped you with the thesis. You must also remember the Head of the Department and the Head of the Institution/Dean.

The page is numbered using lower case Roman numerals. The heading, "ACKNOWLEDGMENTS," is centered and typed in upper case. The text begins a double space below the heading and the page is double-spaced. It should at the end contain the candidate's name.

Abbreviations (Optional)

In writing of the thesis, long word and scientific terms are often used in their abbreviated form.

Therefore, all these abbreviations are listed under a *List of Abbreviations* on a separate page. Inclusion of this page is optional and when present, it is placed after the *Acknowledgments* page. This page is numbered using lower case Roman numerals.

Table of Contents

The Table of Contents is placed immediately after the Acknowledgments or Abbreviations page, if present and lists all the major elements that follow it but should **not** list any item that precedes it. It is constructed on the basis of the final manuscript so that it provides an accurate guide to the text of the thesis. The heading, "TABLE OF CONTENTS," is typed in upper case.

Headings in the Table of Contents are listed as Introduction, etc. It can also be listed as Chapter 1 – Introduction, etc..

Subheadings are optional, but if subheadings are given for one chapter, then subheadings must be given for all other chapters. Headings and sub-headings in the text must correspond exactly in word and form to the Table of Contents. Each subheading level is indented more than the previous with all of the same levels having the same indentation. A reader should be able to see at a glance the number of levels of headings in the Table of Contents.

The page number listed is the first page of each item or section. If a heading in the Table of Contents runs more than one line, it is single-spaced, and the page number is aligned with the bottom line of the heading. A dotted line extends after the last word of each entry to the page number (see appendix).

List of Tables and List of Figures

The Table of Contents is followed by the List of Tables, which is followed by the List of Figures. Each of these begins on a separate page. The heading is centered, between the margins, typed in upper case following the 1 inch top margin. The first entry begins a double space below the heading (see Appendix for an example.)

The List of Tables and the List of Figures include all items of each appropriate category in the thesis. Each title must be presented *exactly* as it is mentioned in the text. If there are numbered tables or figures in the Appendix, these should also be included in the lists. When a table or figure is preceded by a page indicating the number and title of the figure or table (i.e., citation of the figure or table), then the preceding page number is the one listed. Tables and figures should be numbered in the order in which they appear in the thesis.

Tables, Figures and other Illustrations

A ***table*** comprises of any material presented in columnar arrangement, either vertical or horizontal (landscape) anywhere in the thesis. The reader should be able to understand the results given in a table or frame without frequently consulting the text.

Any diagram, drawing, graph, chart, map, photograph, or other type of illustration is designated in the thesis as a ***figure.***

The format of tables may vary with the specialties (disciplines) but must be consistent throughout the thesis. Every table and figure must bear a caption that consists of its number preceded by the word "Table" (e.g. Table 2.3) or "Figure" (e.g. Fig. 3.2) and followed by a descriptive title. When a table or figure is referred to in the text, the reference should be to the table / figure number, "Table 2.3" for example, and not to "the table below."

The location of the title must be the same for all tables/figures—a uniform distance from the top or a uniform distance from the bottom. All tables are captioned at the top and figures at the bottom. In any case, the practice for tables must be consistent for all tables, and the practice for figures must be consistent for all figures within the thesis. ***Arabic numerals*** should be used for tables and figures because most readers have difficulty with a designation such as "Table LVII."

Tables and figures are numbered consecutively throughout the thesis including appendices. The tables and figures of the appendix are identified with capital letters and Arabic numerals (e.g., Table A3 is the third table of Appendix A). Tables and figures are numbered in the order in which they are first mentioned.

Column/row headings must be such as to make the content easily understood by readers. This applies to the legend as well. The legend must also be apt and slick.

Titles of tables and figures may be single-spaced throughout the thesis. The font (typeface) used in tables must be consistent with that used in the text and same margin requirements apply. The font size of the legend can be 2 or 3 points less than the text.

Tables and figures are inserted as soon as possible following their first mention in the text (citation). If a table or figure will not fit on the page where the first reference to it appears, it should be moved to the top of the next page, while filling in the text page with text that would normally come after the table or figure. A table or figure that will fit on a single page must be placed as such and not divided between two pages. If a table or figure is longer than a manuscript page, type "table continues" or "figure continues" in brackets at the bottom right-hand corner of the page.

Tables and figures plus captions must be prepared in a way that preserves thesis margins. If a table or figure needs to be in landscape (positioned sideways), the title must also be sideways with the heading toward the binding edge allowing a proper margin, and the title must be oriented to read with the table or figure. The page number must appear in the usual position.

Oversized tables and figures may be reduced but the table or figure number and title may not be reduced. Tables and figures should be separated from the text (or any other material on the page) and from each other by at least three or four single lines of space.

Figures may be computer generated. When this is not possible, they must be drawn in black waterproof ink. Labels and legends must be typed using the same fonts and size as the text of the paper.

All tables and figures should have title or legend!

Special Materials

Photographs in the thesis may be in colour or in black and white and should be prepared with a background that produces sharp contrast and clear detail. The radiographs (X-rays) must be in black and white. Any photograph, map, or chart smaller than 8¼ x 11½ inches should be mounted on ivory paper (available separately at the stationers).

When photographs are used, they must be clearly reproduced in all copies of the thesis. Large photographs included in a thesis should be printed on photographic or white bond paper. Margin requirements for photographs are the *same* as those for the text of the manuscript. Small photographs may also be mounted using dry-mount procedures or special glue.

If an illustration, figure, map or table is up to two times greater than either dimension of the page, it must be bound in the thesis at the left and folded without the danger of the fold(s) protruding out at the right, top, or bottom being trimmed in the binding process. Materials more than two times greater than either dimension of the page must be inserted in a pocket page, at the end of the thesis in the inside back cover.

As an alternative to mounted photographs, high-quality photocopies of the original photographs may be made directly onto the same paper that is used in the rest of the manuscript. The results are often very good, and the method is less complicated than the processes described.

Chemical Notations and Other Symbols

Symbols, other than letters of the Roman alphabet and Arabic numerals that are not available on a keyboard (these must indeed be rare!), must be drawn carefully and legibly with a fine-pointed pen with black waterproof ink. There should be spacing above, below, and between lines of chemical notation or symbols presented on separate lines to ensure visual clarity. There should be at least *two lines of space* between the subscripts of one line and the superscripts of the line below.

In Microsoft Word, if you click on the 'Insert' key, and then on Symbol, you will see the icon symbols that can be used to insert all sorts of symbols in the text.

Headings and Subheadings

A consistent system of headings must be adopted for use throughout the thesis. Headings indicate the organization of the thesis. Hence, all topics of equal importance have the same level of heading throughout a manuscript (e.g., titles of chapters, headings of sections in a chapter, etc.). The same applies to the sub-headings. Regardless of the number of levels of subheading within a section, they must always follow the same top-down progression.

1. **Chapter heading:** All in capital letters with font size 18 or 20 and bold. The chapter heading should be left aligned. Each new chapter begins on a new page.

   CHAPTER 1

   (Left margin aligned, uppercase, font 18 or 20 and bold heading).

2. **Major heading (section headings)**—should be in font size 14 or 16 and bold and may be underlined, first letter of all major words capitalized. It should be left margin aligned. (Left margin aligned, uppercase, and lowercase, font 14 or 16 and bold heading).
3. **Minor heading (sub-heading level 1 or A)** —should be left margin aligned with font size same as that of text and bold with first letter of all major words capitalized.
4. **Minor division (sub-heading level 2 or B)** —should be of same font size as that of the text, bold and in italics; paragraph heading indented with only first letter of first word capitalized.

Major headings and minor headings and divisions ordinarily do not begin on a new page. Headings should not appear at the bottom of a page with no textual material following. At least two lines of text must follow a heading at the bottom of a page.

References/Bibliographies

It is important to reference your work correctly. If you acknowledge the work of others, you cannot be accused of plagiarizing someone else's work. You also need to give complete details of the item to which you are referring so that readers can easily trace the item whether it is a book chapter, article or webpage. You are also allowing the reader to trace your line of research and to judge its thoroughness.

When gathering information for your thesis from books, journals and web pages it is important that you keep a record of where your information comes from. This can be done by writing down each and every page and article that you have read and webpage that you have visited or by using bibliographic referencing software.

All *theses* should contain appropriate documentation, that is, references to original literature relevant to the research presented in the paper. When quoting scientific research, authors should cite published full papers and avoid reliance on abstracts. The first page of the reference/ bibliography section should immediately follow the last page of the text.

There are many ways of setting out bibliographies and reference lists. Given here is one style—the Vancouver style that is commonly employed in medical and scientific journals.

The referencing of all the material is carried out in two stages. These are:

1. *Citing References in Text*

   When citing in the text, you should use Arabic numerals in superscript or within brackets [e.g.[5] or (5)]; the number in brackets links directly to the *Reference list* at the end of the piece of wcrk (in bibliography or references). There are two ways to include a reference in the text.

   If the author's name naturally forms part of a sentence, then include it exactly as if no reference is being given. Follow the name by a space and the number in the reference list, enclosed in parentheses. (Multiple authorship is dealt with in the same way.) Examples:

   Sharma (2) suggested that ...
   The system developed by Singh and Kapoor (6) is...
   Sahni *et al.* (21) have reported that ...

   (If the number in the brackets is removed, the remaining sentence, including punctuation, must still be correct).

   Multiple references by the same author(s) can be dealt with by placing a **list** of numbers in brackets. Examples:

   Singh (7, 9, 21) has repeatedly argued that ...
   The system developed by Misra and Kumar (7,19) is ...

   If there are two authors, both names should be given in the text. If there are three or more authors, it is permissible (but not obligatory) to use only the name of first author followed by "*et al.*". Note that "*et al.*" is italicized. It is an abbreviation for *et alia* in Latin, meaning "and others".

2. *Reference List at End of Thesis*

There is a distinction between 'References' and 'Bibliography'. References are those sources actually referred to in the text. If " Sharma (3)" occurs in the text, there *must* be a full description of it in the list of references. If there is also a ***bibliography***, then it lists those sources which were consulted and found *relevant,* but are not actually referred to by name in the text. If you use a combined bibliography and list of references, make sure this is clear to the reader.

Only *one single list of references* should be given at the end of the thesis—never one per chapter.

Multiple authors must *never* be reduced to *et al.*, even though they were in the body of the text.

The goal of the list of references must always be *completeness* and *consistency*. Completeness means that from the reference alone (i.e. with no other knowledge of the subject), the reader can locate the original source or obtain a copy.

References should be numbered consecutively ***in the order*** in which they are first mentioned in the text; they should ***not*** be listed alphabetically by author or title or put in date order.

1. Bhansali SK. Gastrointestinal perforations. A study of 96 cases. *J Postgrad Med* 1967;13:1-12.
2. Kishore D, Singh NN, Verma R, Chauhan SS, Verma A, Potluri N, *et al.* Spinal tuberculosis. *J Assoc Physicians India* 2002;50:1332-3.
3. Sharma LK, Gupta S, Soin AS, Sikora SS, Kapoor VK. Generalised peritonitis in India-The tropical spectrum. *Jpn J Surg* 1991;21:272-277.
4. Mathur SR, Dhaiya S, Nayak A, Bhatla N, Singh MK. Sclerosing stromal tumour of ovary—a clinico-

pathological and immunohistochemical study of five cases. *Indian J Pathol Microbiol* 2004;47:333-5.
5. Malhotra R, Singh KD, Bhan S, Dave PK. Primary pyogenic abscess of the psoas muscle. *J Bone Joint Surg Am* 1992;74:278-84.
6. Pathak AK, Bhutani M, Mohan A, Guleria R, Bal S, Kouchupillai V. Non small cell lung cancer (NSCLC): current status and future prospects. *Indian J Chest Dis Allied Sci* 2004;46:191-203.
7. Dewenda NK, Chumber S, Tandon N, Karak AK. Functioning oxyphil adenoma of parathyroid. *J Postgrad Med* 2000;46:215-6.

Note: Do not put brackets (parentheses) around the numbers at the start of each entry in the reference list.

References cited only in tables or figure legends should be numbered in accordance with the sequence established by the first identification in the text of the particular table or figure.

The methods for referencing for other sources are given below:

Printed Publications

Books: You need to give details of the author(s), year of publication, title, edition (if not the 1st), place of publication and publisher.

1. Felig P, Baxter JD. *Endocrinology and Metabolism*. 7th edition. London. Bailliere, Tindall and Cox; 1981.
2. Johnson CD, Taylor I. *Recent Advances in Surgery Vol 23*. Edingburgh: Churchill Livingstone; 2000.

Edited Book

1. Ahuja MS, Kapoor MM. Epidemiological studies on diabetes mellitus in India. In: Ahuja MMS (ed). Epidemiology of Diabetes in Developing countries. New Delhi: Interprint 1979:29-30.

Chapter in Book

1. Daniel W. Foster. Diabetes mellitus. In: *Harrison's Principles of Internal Medicine Vol. 2*. 13th edn. Isselbacher KJ, Braunwald E, Wilson JD, Martin JB, Fauci AS, Kasper DL (eds.); New York, McGraw-Hill Inc 1994; 1979-2000.

Conference Proceedings

1. Anonymous. Proceedings of a consensus development conference on Benign Breast Disease. Breast Disease 1;18-31,2005.
2. Thyroid Research Group. The effect of low dose radioactive iodine ablation of residual thyroid on long term survival. *Hospital Today* 2001;12: 78-82.

Conference Paper

1. Chumber S. Adrenal Function Tests. In: Mohanty BK, Misra SK, Nair A (eds). ENDOCON 2005. Proceedings of the 5th International Endocrine Surgery Conference; 6-10:2005; Puri, Orissa; 2005:39-45.

Government Publications

1. Rajendran R. Oral submucous fibrosis: etiology, pathogenesis, and future research. Bull World Health Organi 1994, 72(6): 985-996.

Dissertations

1. Giridhar V. Effectiveness of different regimens in the treatment of lymphnode tuberculosis: a prospective randomized and follow-up study (dissertation). New Delhi: All India Institute of Medical Sciences; 2003;108.

Dictionary and Similar References

1. Butterworths medical dictionary. 2nd ed. Great Britain: Butterworths; 1978. Gait; p. 703.

Newspaper Article

1. Sharma S. AIIMS gets money wise, hikes charges. Hindustan Times 2005 Nov 29; 1.

Journals

You will find below examples based on the formats used by the ***National Library Medicine*** (NLM) in their database ***Medline***.

Web link.When listing a reference, list all authors if there are 6 or less and the first 6 authors followed by *et al.* If there are more than 6. This is followed by the Title of the article and name of the Journal. The journals should be abbreviated according to the style used by Medline (Web link) (consult the List of Journals Indexed in Index Medicus (Medline)), in the library or check citation on Medline. This is to be followed by the year of the Journal, the volume number and the first and last page. If a journal carries continuous pagination throughout a volume (as many medical journals do) the month and issue number may be omitted.

1. Chinnakotla S, Pande GK, Sahni P, Gupta SD, Maulik M, Kumari R, *et al.* Evaluation of Pringle maneuver during liver resection in a rat model of surgical obstructive jaundice. *J Invest Surg* 2005;18:107-13.
2. Dandona L, Tandon N, Sahni P. Academic medicine and health improvements in India. *Natl Med J India* 2005;18: 53-8.
3. Sharma LK, Sharma A. Cotton-ball phytobezoar simulating oesophageal atresia. *Indian J Pediatr* 1993;60:709-10.
4. Prakash A, Rajalakshmi M, Prasad MR, Anand Kumar TC. Ultrastructural changes in the principal and clear cells in the rat epididymis following the administration of cyproterone acetate. *Indian J Exp Biol* 1979;17:1159-65.
5. Chowdhury UK, Arian B, Talwar S, Kothari SS, Saxena A, Singh R, *et al.* One and one-half ventricle repair: results and concerns. *Ann Thorac Surg* 2005;80:2293-300.

Electronic Publications

1. Ministry of Health. Maternal and Child Health Programme. (Online) Available from URL http://mohfw. nic.in/reports/Yearly % 20 Report % 201995 96/Part-I-6.pdf (accessed on 6 December 2005).

Journal Article in Electronic Format

1. Hudis C. The Latest Thinking in Hormonal Therapy for Breast Cancer in the Adjuvant Setting. Medscape Today (online) 2005 November. Available from URL http://www.medscape.com/viewprogram/4771 (accessed 2005 2 December).
2. Dewenda NK, Chumber S, Tandon N, Karak AK. Functioning oxyphil adenoma of parathyroid. J Postgrad Med [serial online]2000[cited Jan 16];46:215-6. Available from http://www.jpgon-line.com/article.asp.?issn=0022-3859; year = 2000;volume=46;issue=3;s page= 6; aulast = Dewenda.

Appendix

The appendices may contain study proformas, master charts, tables of data, composition of reagents etc. that would otherwise interfere with easy reading of the text. If diverse materials are included, they should be grouped into categories and each category labeled as a separate appendix: Appendix 1, Appendix 2, etc. Each appendix should be titled and listed with its title in the Table of Contents. The appendices follow the reference/ bibliography entries and are paginated continuously.

Binding of Thesis

Cheap, spiral binding of thesis with dirty looking plastic covers should be avoided at all costs.

The entire thesis must be hardbound with leather spine and corners. The title page must be embossed on the hardcover in golden ink. The title page can also be used as a loose paper cover over the hard cover. The colour of the hard cover may be maroon or black. The colour of the thesis submitted by the Master's candidates are maroon in colour. The thesis or dissertation submitted by doctoral candidates are black in colour. The binding can be easily carried out by the local printer and binder.

Remember that a thesis grant that is given to the candidate may be adequately and completely used only for the purposes of a good binding.

The number of copies bound generally depends on the number of guides. Three copies are to be deposited with the Academic Section and each guide should receive one copy. *One copy is retained by the candidate.* Thus the number is **4+x**, where **x** is the number of guides. *Please check if the number is different for your institution.*

Number of copies required = 4+**x**, (where **x** = no. of guides)

The thesis is a valuable publication and one that you will treasure as your *baby* for many years to come. For the next 5 years you will probably refer to it frequently and carry it with you to several interviews as you progress in life. *In fact, most interviews will open with a discussion of your thesis topic!*

Chapter 7

Submission of Thesis

Submission Guidelines

The final submission copies of the thesis or dissertations must be made on approved paper, if your College so requires. The final product should reflect all of these—legible print, readability of format, and uniformity of contrast between paper and print.

Copies of the manuscript must be reproduced on a good photocopying machine or several print-outs must be taken by the candidate. Photocopying must produce sharp, high-contrast copies.

The candidates are generally in a hurry to deposit the copies and hence do not devote the required time for photocopying and binding—they often deposit wet and soggy copies.

All last minutes checks must be performed before depositing the thesis (see Checklist for Candidates).

1. Check pagination: all pages *in each copy* must be in correct order and numbered.
2. Check all diagrams, photos and tables and illustrations.
3. Check bibliography or references
4. Check all preliminary pages are present.
5. Check that abstract page is present.

The thesis in final form, signed by the guides or the thesis committee, must be in the Academic Section/ Registrar's Office by the due date. The thesis is forwarded from the Department through the Head of the Department.

At the time of submission, the student must present the following:

DISSERTATION (MASTER'S)

1. Two deposit copies of the dissertation
2. Two copies of the Thesis Protocol.

THESIS (DOCTORAL)

1. Three deposit copies of the thesis
2. Four copies of Thesis Protocol
3. Four copies of Abstract
4. Actual Thesis read at time of preview
6. Thesis Approval sheet (provided at time of preview).

Thesis/Dissertation Checklist

This checklist may be used by the candidate to ensure that his thesis/dissertation is completed in the proper format without errors. Even the guides should use this checklist before finally signing the thesis prior to submission. A copy of this list may also be used by the college to ensure that the submitted copy of the thesis is complete in all respects.

Checklist for Candidates—see Appendix.

Certificate

The certificate (approval) page must be typed by the student using the same typeface as the text of the paper and printed on approved thesis paper. It will be page ii of the thesis. The certificate page is signed* usually after the final approval of the contents by the guides and all the co-guides. Rarely, the candidate obtains the signature of the guides prior to sending the thesis for binding. **Photocopies of signed approval pages are not acceptable.** For a Doctoral thesis, committee members are to sign all copies after the final defense has been passed.* This is indeed a big moment in your life!

---

* with great flourish and pomp.

Typist/Secretarial Assistant

Most students would type their thesis themselves on a modern computer. The era of typists and typewriters is over. If, for any reason, a student hires a typist to prepare the final copy of the manuscript, the typist should be experienced in typing scholarly papers.

Responsibilities of the student and the typist should be established before typing actually begins so that both parties will have a firm understanding about the work to be performed and the charges to be paid. *The student should allow the typist enough time to work without pressure.* The typist is responsible for preparing a perfect copy of what is presented. The typist should not be required nor be expected to correct errors of spelling, punctuation, or grammar in the manuscript. The manuscript should be given to the typist in correct form, and the typist should be responsible only for typing what the author actually presents.

The student may reasonably expect a typist to work with a typed draft copy and produce a final manuscript of the thesis that meets prescribed standards of margins, spacing, page numbering, and similar matters of format. A typist should not be expected (at least without extra compensation) to perform additional duties such as editing the text, references, or footnotes. Ultimately, it is the student's responsibility to proofread closely for typographical and other errors.

Chapter 8

Copyright and Storage

General Information

When planning to include any information in your thesis or dissertation that you did not create, you have to reference it in the manner already discussed. For some of the information that you may want to include, you are required to obtain permission from authors or such sources that hold a copyright to the above material. You will need this permission irrespective of how you have obtained this information. Permission is required even for the information easily available on the Internet. Even government documents are properties of the Government of India and are not free for reproduction without permission. Permission is also required for using photographs, diagrams or maps. Sometimes, the © symbol on a document is not seen, yet this material may be copyrighted and permission may be required for its use.

Simple quotes from research articles, textbooks, electronic media and Internet may not require copyright permission as this information is clearly cited in the references. However, there is no way of knowing the *limit* to the use of copyright material. This is best resolved by referring to the author(s) of the material or those organizations holding a copyright to such material and seeking their permission for its use. Hence, when in doubt contact the author of the work/holder of rights on the piece you want to use.

Authors or those holding such rights do not deny such permissions when this is required for thesis or dissertations. However, when required for commercial use, you will need clear permission for use of those materials. This may include text, photographs, diagrams, maps, government documents, Internet website material, etc. When using materials that are government property, permission must be sought for their use.

As the author of your thesis or dissertation, you are responsible for obtaining permissions when copyright material has been included in your work. This should be carried out prior to submitting the work to the Dean. However, since this may require additional time. When permissions are not available, such materials should be removed from the thesis or dissertations. All of this is not likely to delay in your appearing for the examinations or for the public defense of dissertation or receiving your degree.

Sometimes, you may change an original copyrighted diagram or chart or text to suit the requirements of your thesis or dissertation. When such an item has been changed significantly, it is considered an *adaptation*. An adaptation is more than the simple change of colour of diagram or font of text. The original concept is still present! Hence, you must give a citation for adapted work too.

You will find a request letter in the appendix that can be used to obtain permission for the use of copyright materials.

Copyright for Your Thesis or Dissertation

Since, copyright is indeed the legal protection of an author's intellectual property—whether literary, audiovisual, or any other creative work, you should include a copyright notice on your thesis as it signals to readers that you acknowledge your legal rights and that you are the copyright owner. It also clearly indicates the year you first published the project in the event of a conflict with any later work. The notice must appear centered on the page

Typical copyright notices take this form:

Copyright by
Neeraj Dewenda 1998
All Rights Reserved.

In order to establish a public record of a thesis and to prevent the unlawful reproduction, use, or distribution of the work, a student may elect to register a copyright. Arrangements for registering a copyright are handled by the college, institution or university. A copyright/registration fee must be paid by the student. Registration establishes a public record of the thesis, the copyright, the author's name and address. Registration is required before the author can file an infringement lawsuit or file for claim of damages.

Storage of Thesis and Dissertations

There are currently no means of storage of thesis and dissertations within the country. Storage of thesis is common as well as compulsory in some countries in the West. Often the designing of the thesis was carried out for purposes of storage by microfilming. However, the era of microfilming is over and nowadays, it would be easier to store thesis on hard-disk, CD or DVD and in other forms in digital format.

There are several sites on the internet where you can access the thesis and dissertations carried out by others for a consideration. Some of these sites will offer to store your thesis for a consideration. *Some sites will also offer to write your thesis for you! So, beware!*

Microfilming

Microfilming of the theses was favoured during the sixties to the eighties. For reproduction of thesis and dissertations on microfilm, the University would create and retains master negatives of the films.

These were available on payment. It is not in vogue now.

Currently, most universities would retain the hard copy along with a CD of your thesis. The candidate must make this available when required.

Chapter 9

Special Issues

Ethical Guidelines for Clinical trials on Human Subjects

In medical specialties, almost all of the theses and dissertations will be carried out on human subjects-men, women, pregnant women, children and special groups- either directly or indirectly. Hence, it is important to be aware of guidelines regarding research in human subjects.

Historical Aspects of Research on Human Subjects

Shocking details of clinical trials on human subjects were revealed during trials of German medical doctors after the Second World War (1939-1945). Most of the research was conducted without consent and invariably exposed all subjects to risk of grave injury if not death. Thus, the Nuremberg Code on ethics of medical research using human subjects was formulated in 1947. Subsequently, the General Assembly of the United Nations adopted the Universal Declaration of Human Rights. In 1964, the World Medical Council formulated general principles on use of human subjects in medical research in addition to specific guidelines for biomedical research–this is known as the Helsinki Declaration. In 1982, the World Health Organization issued the proposal for the international guidelines for biomedical research involving human subjects.

In India, the Indian Council of Medical Research (ICMR), at New Delhi released a policy statement on "Ethical Considerations involved in Research on Human Subjects". This document is being widely used by not only the ICMR but also by other government agencies, research institutions and scientists. This has recently been updated. Included here is a brief discussion on these guidelines.

There is an imperative need of guidelines for research in human subjects. Apart from clinical trials on new drugs, a number of new diagnostic and therapeutic procedures as well as the use of vaccines involve human subjects. The advent of new medical devices, radio-active materials and recombinant DNA products have added a new dimension to the ethical issues involving human subjects. The ushering in of the era of biotechnology, genetic engineering, assisted reproductive techniques, organ transplantation, human gene analysis and gene therapy, medical procedures and therapeutics have undergone tremendous changes. At the same time, these raise several questions of law and ethics that need to be addressed in the new century.

Medical and Related Research on Human Subjects

Medical and other related research in human subjects must ensure that the purpose of research is to increase knowledge about human conditions in relation to their environment. The research must be conducted under such conditions that no person or persons become tools for the betterment of others. Human beings who are subjected to medical research are dealt with in a manner consistent with their dignity and well-being. The research must also be subjected to evaluation at all stages of research design, experimentation, and declaration of results and the ultimate use of results.

It is also imperative that any research using human beings as subjects of medical or scientific research must fulfill the following criteria:

- This research is essential.
- It is voluntary—an informed consent has been obtained.

- It is non-exploitative and guarantees privacy and confidentiality of the participants.
- The research study must employ all precautions and ensure that all steps have been taken to minimize risks to the subjects. The subjects should not suffer any irreversible adverse effects and should (in general) benefit from research.
- The research must at all times be in the hands of professionally qualified scientists and doctors. They should also ensure complete transparency in the process of research and take full responsibility for this.
- The research or experiment and its subsequent application should be used to benefit all human kind.

Ethics and Research

All research involving human subjects should be conducted in accordance with the four basic ethical principles, namely *autonomy* (respect for person/subject) *beneficence*, *non-maleficence* (do no harm) and *justice*.

The Principal Investigator is the person responsible for not only undertaking research but also for observance of the rights, health and welfare of the subjects recruited for the study. It is mandatory that all proposals on biomedical research involving human subjects should be cleared by an appropriately constituted Institutional Ethics Committee (IEC) or Institutional Review Board (IRB).

Special guidelines exist for including pregnant or nursing women, research related to termination of pregnancy, research related to pre-natal diagnostic techniques, children and vulnerable groups, viz. persons who are economically or socially disadvantaged, mentally challenged persons and prisoners, students, subordinates, employees, service personnel etc. who have reduced autonomy as research subjects.

Informed Consent: For all biomedical research involving human subjects, the investigator must obtain the informed consent of the prospective subject or in the case of an individual who is not capable of giving informed consent, the consent of a legal guardian.

Compensation for participation: Subjects may be paid for the inconvenience and time spent and should be reimbursed for expenses incurred, in connection with their participation in research. This may not be possible for a thesis or other unfunded research, but these subjects may receive free medical services.

Clinical Evaluation of Drugs and Vaccines

Sometimes, it is essential to carry out research on human subjects to discover better medical and therapeutic modalities for the benefit of mankind. It is also clear that such research on normal subjects and patients is associated with some degree of risk to the individual concerned. These guidelines have been framed to carry out the evaluation of drugs, vaccines, devices and other diagnostic materials on human subjects including herbal remedies, in accordance with the basic ethical principles. These guidelines are important for the protection of research subjects against any avoidable risk and to guide the researchers in the preparation of research proposals/protocols.

Clinical trial of drugs are randomized single— or double—blind controlled trials in human subjects, designed to evaluate prospectively the safety and effectiveness of new drugs/new formulations. The drug is usually tested through clinical trials in four phases. The first three of the following four phases of clinical trials of drug require ethical clearance:

Phase I: The objective of a phase I clinical trial is to determine the safety of the maximum tolerated dose in healthy adults of both sexes.

Phase II: These are controlled studies conducted in a limited number of patients of both sexes to determine therapeutic uses, effective dose range and further evaluation of safety and pharmacokinetics when necessary. These studies are usually limited to 3-4 centres.

Phase III: The purpose of these trials is to obtain adequate data about the efficacy and safety of drugs in a larger number of patients of both sexes in multiple centres, usually in comparison with a standard drug and/or a placebo. On successful completion of phase III trials, permission is granted for marketing of the drug.

Phase IV: After approval of the drug for marketing, phase IV study or post marketing surveillance is undertaken to obtain additional information about the drug's risks, benefits and optimal use. Although this is outside the purview of the ethical committee, it is an important aspect of drug trial on the long-term effects of the drugs and the adverse reactions induced by drugs, if any, should be brought to the notice of the Ethics Committee.

Trials on vaccines are usually conducted in three phases.

Research in Human Genetics

In no other area of biomedical research has there been a greater concern for ethical issues than in the field of human genetics. In recent years, this concern has grown even further because of the possibility of *commercial* eugenics. With the completion of the *Human Genome Project*, there is an urgent need for clear-cut guidelines and dissemination of information to all. Serious issues related to participation of human subjects in genetic research are raised particularly when the intervention involves rights of human embryo and subjects who are not competent to give informed consent.

Clinical research in fields of human genetics and human genome, gene therapy must be subject to general ethical principles of being voluntary and of protection from harm. Research in these areas must take into account the following:

1. The harm may not only be physical, but also psychosocial.
2. There is great importance of spoken word in medical genetics, since genetic counselling is akin to therapy in other fields.
3. Genetic counselling deals with discussion on personal matters such as reproductive options, and the couple may have to make a choice with far reaching social implications.
4. Genetic manipulations have consequences for the future, some of which are unknown.
5. There is greater likelihood of situations cropping up where there is conflict of interest between an individual, and that of family and society at large.
6. The Institutional Ethical Committees reviewing research proposals related to research on human genetics should have necessary expertise, which includes knowledge of latest developments in the field of human genetics.
7. There must be strict guidelines as well as control of local Governments to prevent the misuse of genetic tests and other therapeutics that may arise from this testing.

Guidelines for use of Laboratory Animals in Research

Laboratory animals used in medical colleges play a vital role in teaching and research. The animal is used as a substitute for man as most laboratory animals have the same or similar anatomical and physiological features. Animal experiments give an insight to the students about the etiology, diagnosis, progression and methods of prevention of various diseases. Commonly used animals in medical colleges are frogs, rats, mice, rabbits, guinea pigs, cats, dogs, monkeys and to lesser extent sheep.

It is obligatory on the part of Investigators/ students to handle the animals gently, following the guidelines of ethical consideration for animal use. In India, such guidelines have been devised by the Indian Council of Medical Research and Indian National Science Academy, New Delhi. Such guidelines provide the basic minimum provisions for animal care in medical colleges or other research centers using animals for teaching or research purposes.

According to the Medical Council of India requirement, it is mandatory to have animal facilities attached to every teaching medical college. The various species of animals required for medical colleges should be procured from recognized sources. Medical Colleges should procure the breeding stock from a reliable source for initiating a colony. The following must be adhered to during use of animals:

a. *Food and Water:* Good quality *feed* and water should be provided *ad libitum* to animals that should be fed palatable, non-contaminated, and nutritionally adequate food. Watering devices, such as drinking tubes should be examined routinely to ensure their proper operation. There should be minimum contamination by urine and faeces.
b. *Sanitation and cleanliness:* Animal rooms, corridors, storage spaces, and other areas should be cleaned regularly. Soiled litter material should be removed routinely. Animal cages, racks and accessory equipment, such as feeders and watering devices, should be washed and cleaned frequently to keep them free from contamination.
c. *Veterinary care:* Wherever required, adequate veterinary care must be provided under the supervision and guidance of a registered veterinarian or a person trained and experienced in laboratory animal sciences. Diseased animals should be isolated from healthy ones.
d. *Personnel hygiene and training of staff:* Initial in-house training should be imparted to the staff associated with animal facility along with protec-

tive gears (gloves, masks, head cover, coat, shoes, etc.)

e. *Surgical procedures and duration of experiment:* Multiple surgical procedures on an animal for any experiment are not to be practiced unless specified in a protocol.
f. *Record keeping:* Record maintenance should be strict in the Animal Facilities. This includes data on staff, items on stock, animal stock procurement and supply, records of experiments or procedures conducted with the number of animals used in each experiment, clinical record of sick animals and any treatment administered and morbidity and mortality record.
g. *Anesthesia and Euthanasia:* The scientists should ensure that the procedures which are considered painful are conducted under appropriate anesthesia as recommended for each species of animals. It must also be ensured that the anesthesia is administered to sustain for the full duration of experiment and at no stage the animal is conscious to perceive pain during the experiment. In the event of a decision to *euthanise* an animal on termination of an experiment or otherwise, an approved method of euthanasia should be adopted and the investigator must ensure that the animal is clinically dead before it is sent for disposal. Carcasses should be disposed off either by incineration or deep burial method. The procedure should be carried out quickly and painlessly in an atmosphere free from fear or anxiety. The choice of a method will depend on the nature of study, the species of animal and number of animals to be sacrificed.
h. *Animal houses:* should be properly constructed and well maintained.
i. *Budgeting:* To maintain a proper animal house, adequate budgeting should be done in the general budget of the medical college or research organization. This should include salaries for the staff, plan and non-plan expen-

ditures. If the medical college is maintaining the animal house for breeding purposes also, then the expenditure is much more than if the college is procuring the animals.

Approval of Ethical Committee

Ethical committees are standing committees of all universities and institutions and are appointed by the head of the Institution or University. They are headed by persons who are independent of the institution or university. The Dean of the Institution or a person of similar stature is coordinator for this committee.

Approval of Ethical committee should be sought for research proposals that are clinical trials involving animal or human subjects that may cause pain or place the patient to experience a compromise in bodily function, trials of newer drugs or vaccines, that may modify the presentation, course or outcome of the disease, a new surgical procedure or modifications of an old surgical procedure.

Effectively, this implies that ideally all research protocols should be submitted to the Ethical Committees for approval.

Such approvals also enhance the value of research papers when submitted to specific journals for publications.

After obtaining the signatures of all the guides, the research protocol is submitted through the Head of the Department prior to the date of the meeting of the Ethical Committee. The proposals are discussed at the meeting and a report is submitted to the guide of the research protocol with clear directions of approval, disapproval or those for modifications.

When required, the research protocol has to be resubmitted after the modifications suggested by the Ethical Committee have been incorporated into the protocol.

The research protocol can be pursued while awaiting the final approval of the Ethical Committee.

Rejection of a Thesis Protocol

Proposals for research are generally not rejected. Sometimes, the Faculty of the department will suggest modifications to be incorporated in the research protocol. Rarely, some of the suggestions render a protocol unfit to be followed - usually an outcome of a too hasty submission without adequate brain-storming. Such research protocols can be easily modified and resubmitted for approval.

Rejection of a Thesis or Dissertation

Once the thesis is submitted to the Dean, it is forwarded to two or three External Examiners for evaluation and approval of the thesis or dissertation.

Often, the institution or university will provide guidelines for assessment and approval of the thesis or dissertation.

A thesis or dissertation may be rejected and sent back to the guide and candidate if it does not meet the specified guidelines or carries too many mistakes.

The examiner should provide a detailed list of the reasons of rejection. This should be made available to the guide and candidate for corrections and modifications.

Reasons for Rejection of Thesis

Spelling mistakes, severe grammatical errors, wrong referencing, incorrect analysis of data and incorrect interpretation of results are the reasons for rejection of a thesis. Of those listed above, the first three are the causes in 99 out of 100 *theses* returned or rejected—and all of these should have been corrected even before submission of the thesis and often, it is the candidate who has foolishly not complied with the instructions of the guides in carrying out the corrections.

This is a moment of recriminations but it must also be realized that this is the only time available with the candidate for correction of mistakes. These must be carried out without a moments delay. Once such modifications or corrections have been incorporated in the text, the thesis is re-submitted to the same examiner for re-evaluation and final approval.

Misconduct in Research

The academic freedom that the students and faculty enjoy in a college, institution or university comes with added responsibility of honesty and trust in research. Hence, every institution expects the highest standards of professional and ethical conduct in all areas of research and all related activities and specifically in thesis and dissertation.

Any allegation of misconduct that may arise in the above settings must be expeditiously resolved in a fair manner using such guidelines that safeguard the interests of all concerned parties.

Since misconduct may occur in the shadow of ignorance of all aspects of the defined policies relating to research and writing of thesis and dissertations, all institutions and universities are *duty bound* to make available such guidelines to all those engaged in research. This is the first and the most important step in prevention of misconduct in research.

Misconduct in research is any action that is intended to deceive or defraud. This may include fabrication of spurious data, omission of data, selective reporting, misappropriation of intellectual property (i.e. research plans or data of others) and false accusations. Mistreatment of animals and human subjects too is misconduct. Other forms of misconduct include:

a. Falsification of data.
b. Plagiarism-appropriating another author's works without consent or correct documentation.

c. Conflict of interests when representing two different parties.
d. Fraud and misrepresentation in deceiving others to secure unfair advantages.
e. Non-compliance of set and defined regulations.
f. Misappropriation of research funds.

It is pertinent to mention that *honest error or honest differences in interpretation of data is not misconduct*.

Methodology in Enquiry

On a written complaint of misconduct, an independent standing Enquiry Committee appointed by the Dean / Director of the Institution or University conducts an enquiry as per defined guidelines.

In an immediate meeting, the accused and accuser are questioned independently by the Enquiry Committee. All parties are excused while the Enquiry Committee deliberates on the need of a full enquiry on the basis of available information.

On completion of investigations, the Enquiry Committee reports to the Dean/Director/Disciplinary Committee about its findings and whether misconduct has occurred and makes recommendations for action. The Head of the Institution will communicate to the accused at the earliest in writing and give him/her time to file a reply. A final decision is taken only after this reply is received or the defined time has lapsed.

All proceedings remain confidential and all records are sealed. On completion of the review process, a report is conveyed to all parties whether involved directly or indirectly. The Institution will also undertake all efforts to preserve and restore the dignity and reputations of all persons alleged to have been engaged in research when such allegations are incorrect or unsubstantiated. *The exoneration of all parties will be in writing.*

When research funds are involved, the Dean will impound all such accounts and on completion of enquiry such funding agencies will be informed in writing about the results and to take proper consequent action or make available such funds for further research.

Assessment of a Thesis/Dissertation

This is a small note for the Faculty members who are in the process of assessing a thesis or dissertation. Some Universities may make available to examiners some form of guidelines, but often there are no strict guidelines for assessment of the thesis or dissertation. Many examiners would have over the years evolved their own criteria for assessment of thesis/dissertation. Some are so stringent, that they always send the thesis back for review or corrections or rewriting!

The purpose of this note is to create uniformity in the process of assessment of a thesis or dissertation. Of course, the thesis is assessed at the time of Public Defense in the open forum, but this is not true for the dissertation. It always rests on the *mercy* of the Examiner.

The aim of the thesis/dissertation is to assess a student's ability to analyse a large body of material, organise it, and write it up in a manner that sustains a persuasive argument. The requirement is not to produce original work (*no thesis has won the Nobel Prize*) but it is to write a piece of research that demonstrates a strong capacity for independent thought (*most Nobel Prize winners have written one!*).

Chapter **10**

Appendices

Appendix 1: Sample of Title Page–Master's Degree

TITLE OF THE DISSERTATION
(ALL IN CAPITAL LETTERS)

Thesis

Submitted to the Faculty of

____

in Partial Fulfillment of the

Requirements for the

Degree of Master of Surgery (General Surgery)

Place of submission,
Month/year of submission (Your Full Name)

(This page does not carry a page number)
(This title page should also be the front cover/outer jacket of the hard-bound thesis)

Appendix 2: Sample of The Thesis/ Certificate Page

TITLE OF THE THESIS
(ALL IN CAPITAL LETTERS)

Thesis

Submitted to the

All India Institute of Medical Sciences

for the Degree of

Doctor of Philosophy
in
Microbiology

Approved:

Dr. (type name), Department of Microbiology,
All India Institute of Medical Sciences
New Delhi.

Dr. (type name), Department of Microbiology,
Guru TegBahadur Medical College,
New Delhi.

Dr. (type name), Department of Pathology,
Vardhman Mahavir Medical College and
Safdarjung Hospital
New Delhi.

Dr. (type name), Department of Surgery,
Maulana Azad Medical College
New Delhi.

Dr. (type name), Department of Microbiology,
Lady Hardinge Medical College,
New Delhi.

Month/year of graduation at which degree is conferred

Full Name of Student

Appendix 3: Sample of Certificate (Approval) Page

CERTIFICATE

This is to certify that the subject matter of the thesis entitled–"Typhoidal perforation of the Intestine" is the result of the original work undertaken by Dr. Vinay Kumar Rai under our supervision.

Dr. (type name), Professor, Department of (Type here), College (Type here), Place (Type here)

Dr. (type name), Professor, Department of (Type here), College (Type here). Place (Type here)

Dr. (type name), Professor, Department of (Type here), College (Type here). Place (Type here)

Dr. (type name), Professor, Department of (Type here), College (Type here), Place (Type here)

(To be typed by the student)

Appendix 4: Sample of Dedications Page

DEDICATION

Dedicated to K.D. Singh
untimely death on 11th Nov. 1987.

Appendix 5: Sample of Acknowledgements Page

ACKNOWLEDGEMENTS

I would like to express my sincere gratitude to Dr. Sunil Chumber for his continuous support and guidance in the conduct of this work, from its inception to the conclusion. His advice has been invaluable in tackling the difficulties and in the final presentation of the thesis in its current form.

Dr. Nikhil Tandon has been a source of much-needed advice as well as patients referred from the Department of Endocrinology for surgery to our unit. His meticulous review of the thesis has helped me present this work in a much better form than would have been possible otherwise.

I would also like to express my heartfelt thanks to Dr. Anurag Srivastava for his invaluable help in getting this work completed on time. Statistical analysis of the data seemed a frightful proposition till he showed how. I am grateful to him for giving me the benefit of his experience, his time and his computer in the completion of this work.

I am indebted to all my friends and colleagues in Unit I, Department of Surgery for extending their full support in the conduct of the thesis as well as for their cooperation in allowing me time for its completion.

The unflinching and unconditional support that I have received from my parents cannot be over-emphasized. I cannot thank them enough.

Lastly, I would like to thank all the patients who were a part of this study for placing their trust in this work. I hope they shall find their trust justified.

AIIMS, New Delhi **Dr. Rachit Gupta**
June, 2001

Appendix 6: Sample of Table of Contents

TABLE OF CONTENTS

iii

Appendix 7: Sample of List of Tables Pages

LIST OF TABLES

iv

(Typed on a separate page)

Appendix 8: Sample of List of Figures Page

LIST OF FIGURES

FIGURE PAGE

v

(Typed on a separate page)

Appendix 9: Sample of Introduction Page

INTRODUCTION

This is the first chapter of the thesis. A candidate is expected to bring out the necessity of undertaking the research that is being reported in the thesis. For this purpose the candidate should give a brief account of the background information and then point out the missing link (which is normally the work carried out by the candidate).

Appendix 10: Sample of Aims and Objectives Page

AIIMS AND OBJECTIVES

The aim of the present study was to investigate the presence of an alternate promotor within the first *intron* of human *cathepsin L gene* that is responsible for the transcription of *h cAT LB*.

For this purpose, following objectives were undertaken:

1. To determine whether first *intron* contains a functionally active *promotor.*
2. To identify the minimal *promotor region* by deletion analysis.
3. To identify functionally active *transcription factor binding motifs* in this *promotor.*

Appendix 11: Sample of Review of Literature Page

REVIEW OF LITERATURE

In this section, some students include literature, which is remotely related to the work in order to make thesis bulky. This kind of exercise does not serve any purpose. Therefore, you should only cite relevant literature in this section.

Appendix 12: Sample of Materials and Methods Page

MATERIALS AND METHODS

Materials

In this section, the candidate should give a list of all chemical, reagents and other materials used in the study along with their source (name of company, city, country). Reagents received as *gratis* should also be mentioned in this section.

Methods

Description of the methods should be such that by following your description the reader may be able to perform the experiment. The name, the make (Model no. and source of instruments should be mentioned wherever they first appear in the methodology.

A brief account of the statistical methods used for the analysis of results may also be mentioned in this section.

Appendix 13: Sample of Results and Analysis Page

RESULTS AND ANALYSIS

It may be advisable to very briefly describe the rationale of performing an experiment in the beginning of each part before you describe your results. Also while describing your results it may help the readers to understand them if you pinpoint the piece of information in figures by making a mention of the line number, arrow etc. in citation.

Appendix 14: Sample of Discussion Page

DISCUSSION

In this section you are expected to discuss your results in the light of all existing literature. This may include justification of the methodology used, corroborating your findings by the previous reports etc. Also you should highlight in what way your study has contributed to the already existing knowledge in the field. Some universities and academic institutions permit combining this section with the results under Results and Discussion.

Appendix 15: Sample of Conclusions Page

CONCLUSIONS

Conclusions of your findings should be drawn in the light of the existing literature. In case your conclusions are at variance with the known facts, they should either be supported by your experimental data or you should offer a plausible explanation.

Appendix 16: Sample of Summary Page

SUMMARY

The purpose of this section is to briefly describe your thesis.

The summary of the thesis should be such that the reader could get a reasonably good idea of the work just by reading this section. Therefore, you should give a brief introduction of your work in 3 to 4 lines followed by the salient points of the study. The summary should not exceed 2 pages.

Appendix 17: Sample of References/Bibliography Page

REFERENCES/BIBLIOGRAPHY

It is often observed that some references given in the text are not listed in this section and some references given here are not included in the text.

References appearing in the legend to a figure or table are most often overlooked. Similarly, when a portion of text is deleted from final (or nearly final) version of the text after the bibliography section has been completed, usually references contained in this portion are not deleted from the list. Therefore, it is advisable that a candidate should make list of references from the text after it has been finalized and tally it with reference section.

Appendix 18: Sample of Appendix Page

APPENDIX

Important information not incorporated in the main body of the text to avoid discontinuity is included in this section. In basic sciences disciplines, it mainly contains the composition of reagents used in the study. However, composition of commonly used reagents need not be mentioned. The information in this section need not be descriptive.

Appendix 19

Cut along this line

Protocol Submission Checklist

Student's Name: ______________________

Department : ______________________

Check off that you have complied with the items below and obtain signatures of Guides before submission of your Thesis/Dissertation protocol.

Title Page/Signature Page

- ☐ Title page contains the complete title of the research protocol.
- ☐ Title page contains correct names and correct designations of all guides.
- ☐ All guides have signed the research protocol.

Introduction

- ☐ The introduction is brief
- ☐ It clearly introduces the research problem.

Aims and objectives

- ☐ Is the aim of the research protocol defined?
- ☐ Are there too many aims?
- ☐ Are the objectives clear and defined?
- ☐ Are there too many objectives that you are trying to achieve?
- ☐ Have you reflected on each of the above carefully?

Materials and Methods

- ☐ Is the defined methodology attached?
- ☐ Is the number of patients or cases or experiments clearly defined?
- ☐ Are the numbers achievable in the set time?
- ☐ Ethical Committee clearance is obtained.
- ☐ Funding agency clearance has been obtained, if required.

Review of Literature

- ☐ Has the relevant material been reviewed?
- ☐ Is the review adequate?

References

- ☐ Only one consistent style is followed for referencing.
- ☐ Does not contain too many references.
- ☐ Does not contain too many old references.

Others

- ☐ Is it possible to complete this thesis/dissertation on time.

Appendix 20

Cut along this line

Thesis Submission Checklist

Student's Name: ____________________

Department: ____________________

Check off that you have complied with the items below:

1. **Abstract Page (required for all Master's and Doctoral students)**
   - ☐ The heading on the page includes the title of the thesis and 'abstract'.
   - ☐ The text is single spaced and not more than 300 words.
2. **Title Page/ Certificate Page**
   - ☐ Correct names of students, guides and destinations are listed.
   - ☐ Space for signatures of all guides on the title page is adequate.
   - ☐ Sentence capitalization is used for the title and proper nouns.
3. **Dedication**
   - ☐ Dedication begins on a new page.
4. **Acknowledgements**
   - ☐ Acknowledgements begin on a new page.
5. **Table of Contents**
   - ☐ Headings match text exactly in wording, capitalization, and listed page numbers.
   - ☐ Page numbers listed are right justified.
6. **All Chapters**
   - ☐ Does the first page of each chapter begin 2" from the top of the page?
   - ☐ Is the text double-spaced?
   - ☐ Are paragraphs indented consistently throughout the text?
   - ☐ Are abbreviations consistent throughout the text?
   - ☐ Page numbers in Arabic numerals without additional punctuations.
7. **Thesis Form and Format**
   - ☐ Margins on each page are at least 1" at the top, 1½" on the left, at least 1" at the right and 1¼" at the bottom.
   - ☐ Page numbers are a) centered below the text, b) in the same font as the text, and c) 1" from the bottom of the page to the top of the number.
   - ☐ All pages are numbered (except title page).

- ☐ Main chapter headings are left-aligned and in all capital letters.
- ☐ Lower level headings are formatted consistently for each level.
- ☐ All pages contain text, diagrams, tables and figures.
- ☐ No heading is present at the bottom of a page unless at least four lines of text follow it.
- ☐ No text of just one line or less appears alone on the last page of a chapter.

8. **Tables and Figures (Graphs, Photographs, etc.)**
   - ☐ A consistent style is used for tables and figures throughout the thesis.
   - ☐ Figures and tables placed landscape (side-ways) on the page have top at binding edge.
   - ☐ Table captions are at the top of the tables; figure captions are beneath the figures.
   - ☐ Capitalization, punctuation, and format of table and figure captions are consistent throughout.
   - ☐ Numerical data in tables are lined up by decimal place; column headings are centered above columns of numbers.
   - ☐ Table notes are placed beneath the bottom table line.
9. **Appendices**
   - ☐ Main headings are formatted like main headings in the text.
   - ☐ Each appendix page is numbered in the same manner as text pages.
10. **Copyright Page**
    - ☐ Does your name appear exactly as it does on the title page.
11. **References**
    - ☐ Only one consistent style is used throughout the submitted thesis or dissertation.
12. **Final Assessment**
    - ☐ The Guide has reviewed this thesis or dissertation and it is complete and ready for submission.
    - ☐ The candidate must indicate that he/she has made all corrections as advised by all guides.

(Signature of Candidate)	**(Signature of Guide)**

Appendix 21

COPYRIGHT PERMISSION LETTER

Name of Candidate ....
Name of Degree...
Name of College / University or Institute..................................

This letter e authorizes Dr. / Mr./Ms......................................
(name of candidate) to use..
....
(complete description of material or citation of the original material) as part of his/her thesis / dissertation for the partial requirements of ....
(name of degree) at ....
(name of college or university).

- ☐ This permission also extends to future revisions and editions of the thesis / dissertation.
- ☐ This permission also extends to non-commercial publication and future revisions of such publications.
- ☐ This permission also extends to commercial publication and future revisions of such publications.
- ☐ Permission is also granted to other colleges or publishers that intend to copy and distribute the thesis or dissertation either in print or electronically.

Name of copyright holder..

Title ....

Signature Date..

Company ....

[Your signing of this letter will also confirm that you own (or your company owns) the copyright to the above-described material.]

Appendix 22

CHECKLIST FOR ASSESSMENT OF THESIS/DISSERTATION

The following is a checklist that may be used for assessing a thesis or dissertation.

Checklist for assessment of a thesis/dissertation

- ☐ The thesis meets the set criteria for uniformity in manuscript.
- ☐ Correct designing of the research question.
- ☐ Correct methodology has been followed.
- ☐ Correct results have been reached.
- ☐ Correct conclusions have been drawn.
- ☐ Adequate amount of hours have been devoted to the work.
- ☐ Meet the objectives which should be set out at the beginning.
- ☐ Sustains a coherent and well-developed argument.
- ☐ Presented in a scholarly manner.
- ☐ On successful completion, does the student benefit in the following manner:
  - develops an expertise in their specialist area of study
  - develops analytical capacities
  - develops ability to express his/her ideas on paper
  - develops research skills.

Chapter 11

Bibliography and References

Following is a listing of style manuals approved for use in writing theses. Most formats are available on the Internet. There are no recommended Indian sites. It is suggested that while writing your thesis, *only one style may be followed.*

Bibliography and References

1. *Style Manual for Guidance in the Preparation of Papers for Journal*, 3rd edition. New York: American Institute of Physics, 1978.
2. *Publication Manual,* 5th edition. Washington, DC: American Psychological Association, 2001.
3. *American Sociological Association Style Guide*, 2nd edition. Washington, DC: American Sociological Association, 1997.
4. *Chicago Manual of Style*, 14th edition. Chicago: University of Chicago, 1993.
5. *Scientific Style and Format*, 6th edition. Cambridge, UK: Cambridge University Press, 1994.
6. Dodd, Janet, Ed. *The ACS Style Guide, A Manual for Authors and Editors,* 2nd edition. Washington, 1997.
7. Gilbaldi, Joseph. *MLA Handbook for Writers of Research Papers*, 6th edition. New York: The Modern Language Association of America, 2003.
8. Slade, Carole, Campbell, William, and Ballou, Stephen. *Form and Style,* 10th edition. Boston: Houghton Mifflin Company, 1997.
9. Turabian, Kate L. *A Manual for Writers of Term Papers, Theses, and Dissertations*, 6th edition. Chicago: University of Chicago Press, 1996.
10. Writing the Winning Dissertation: A Step by Step Guide by Allan A. Glatthorn.
11. Writing Your Dissertation in Fifteen minutes a Day: A Guide to Starting, Revising and Finishing Your Doctoral Thesis by Joan Bolker.
12. Dissertations and Theses from start to Finish by John D. Cone, Sharon L. Foster.
13. Theses and Dissertations: A Guide to Planning , Research and Writing by R. Murray Thomas, Dale L. Brubaker.
14. Secrets for a successful dissertation by Jacqueline Fitzpatrick, Jan Secrist, Debra J. Wright.

15. The Clockwork Muse: A Practical Guide to writing Theses, Dissertations and Books by Eviatar Zerubavel.
16. Surving your Dissertation: A comprehensive Guide to content and process by Kjell Erik Rudestam, Rae R. Newton.
17. Writing and Publishing Your Thesis, Dissertation and Research by P. Paul Heppner and Mary J. Heppner.
18. Writing a Thesis: Substance and Style by R. Keith Van Wagenen.
19. Moses L (1985), "Statistical Concepts Fundamental to Investigations," The New England Journal of Medicine, 312, 890- 897. Pocock S (1983), Clinical Trials, New York: John Wiley & Sons.
20. Dallal GE Some Aspects of Study Design. URL http://www.tufts.edu/~gdallal/STUDY.HTM (last accessed 8.5.2006).
21. Levine SJ. Writing and Presenting Your Thesis or Dissertation. URL http://www.learnerassociates.net/dissthes/ (Last accessed On 1 March 2006).
22. Thesis Handbook at (http://www.tele.sunyit.edu/ThesisHandbook.html).
23. How to write a Dissertation or Bedtime Reading for People Who Do Not Have Time to Sleep at (http://www.cs.purdue.edu/homes/dec/essay. dissertation. html).
24. Experimental Digital Library of M.I.T. Theses at (http://theses.mit.edu/).
25. How to Be a Good Graduate Student/ Advisor at (http://www.cs.indiana.edu/how.2b/how.2b.html).
26. How to Organize your Thesis at (http://www. sce.carleton.ca/faculty/chinneck/thesis.html).
27. Pepperdine University's Graduate School at (http://gsep.pepperdine.edu/studentservices/dissertation/education/).
28. Checklist is also available from the Graduate School Thesis/Dissertation Preparation Guide (accessed on 2.12.2005) available from URL: http://academics. memphis.edu/gradschool/tdinfo.html).
29. Ethical considerations involved in research on human subjects, Indian Council of Medical Research (ICMR), 2000, New Delhi.
30. Guidelines for medical research in animals, ICMR, 2001, New Delhi.
31. Guidelines for care and use of animals in scientific research, Indian National Science Academy, First Edition: 1992 , Revised Edition: 2000, New Delhi.
32. 9.11 Misconduct in Research: Academic affairs policies and procedures manual. Florida International University. Available at URL http://www.fiu.edu/ugs thesis_dissertation_ manual.html accessed on 3.3.2006.

Index

F

G

H

L

M

O

P

R

S

T